Metabolic Syndrome Survival Guide

Learn to Prevent Diabetes
and
Heart Attack

D0483785

Mariam Manoukian, MD, PhD

Jerry Manoukian, MD

WESTCHESTER
PUBLISHING COMPANY

Los Altos, California

We have taken every effort to ensure that the information and recommendations presented in this book are in accord with current medical knowledge and standard of care at time of publication. Our understanding of Metabolic Syndrome and of medicine in general is constantly evolving. This book complements, but is not a substitute for, the physician-patient relationship. The authors, editors and publisher cannot accept any responsibility for errors or omissions or for consequences from application of the information in this book, and make no warrants, express or implied, with respect to its contents.

Library of Congress Control Number 2004103068

Copyright © 2004 by Mariam Manoukian, MD, PhD, and Jerry Manoukian, MD

Manufactured in the United States of America. All rights reserved. No portion of this material may be reproduced in any form or by any means without written permission of the authors.

7   6   5   4   3   2

International Standard Book Number 0-917010-75-2

To obtain copies of this book, contact
Manoukian Medical Group
2500 Hospital Drive, Building 4
Mountain View, CA 94040

www.manoukian.org

Westchester Publishing Company
342 State Street, Suite 4
Los Altos, CA 94022

Metabolic Syndrome
Survival Guide

Preface

This book was inspired by our patients and was written for them. Day after day in the office we are asked the same questions, "Why did I get diabetes?" "What are my chances?" "What should I eat?" "What should my cholesterol be?" "How much should I exercise?" and so on. We thought a book describing all of these conditions would become very handy. This book is our answer to questions, hopefully something like a reference guide for the patients, actually for just anybody. Medical science moves forward with great jumps, and writing a book like this was challenging for two practicing physicians, because every couple of months there is something new that needed to be included in the book. We tried to do our best.

We would like to hear your comments and questions, and certainly we will include the answers in the second edition. You can reach us at www.manoukian.org

ACKNOWLEDGEMENTS

We want to thank
  Our children, parents and family for unfailing support and love.
  Our patients for everything they teach us.

Karen Hoxeng, our masterful editor, whose concentration and focus is exceeded only by her charm.

Richard Kharibian, who designed the pages and the cover and did the layout that transformed the book into something visually pleasing.

Rusan Sarian, for generously giving us the privilege of sharing the *Still Life* art for the cover. It was painted by her grandfather, famous Armenian painter, Martiros Sarian.

Our daughter, Elize, for her creative imagination and for allowing us to publish her poem.

Our talented sisters-in-law, Nune Markosyan and Sona Arabian, for their wonderful digital artwork used in the book.

Our teachers, valued colleagues, and friends, Drs Lawrence Crapo and Frederick St Goar, for their extensive review, encouragement and valuable comments.

Dr Gerald Reaven, for developing the concept of Syndrome X. His and other researchers' tireless efforts are the basis for this book.

About the Authors

Mariam and Jerry Manoukian live and practice medicine together in the heart of Silicon Valley.

Mariam Avakian Manoukian was born and raised in Soviet Armenia. She attended the Yerevan Medical Institute and completed postdoctoral training in endocrinology at the All Union Institute of Endocrinology in Moscow, where she earned her PhD in neuroendocrinology (diseases related to the pituitary hormones). Her first book, *ABCs of Diabetes,* was published in Armenian in 1990. After moving to the US in 1992, she completed her residency in internal medicine at Santa Clara Valley Medical Center in San Jose, California. She is board certified in internal medicine and lectures about Metabolic Syndrome to physicians and other health professionals. Her practice spans internal medicine, endocrinology and primary care.

Dr Jerry was raised in California and attended medical school at Hahnemann University in Philadelphia. He completed residency training in internal medicine at Santa Clara Valley Medical Center. He lectures on the potential interactions of herbal remedies and prescribed medication. His practice includes internal medicine and primary care.

They have two fast-growing children, Elize and Greg, from whom they've learned most of the important stuff, how to love and how to play.

Contents

Introduction

WHY YOU NEED TO KNOW ABOUT METABOLIC SYNDROME

Progress is the mother of problems.
—G.K. Chesterton

Diabetes is a common disease and incidence is increasing worldwide. About 8% of the population, or 17 million people, have diabetes in the United States. 5.4 million of these people are unaware they have it. Each year 798,000 Americans develop diabetes, translating to 2200 each day. This is largely fueled by the epidemic of obesity, where 60% of Americans are overweight and about 19% are obese. Obesity is the unnatural, but logical, consequence of the technological progress bringing us fast food, large quantities of sugared beverages, and inactivity.

This book is about Metabolic Syndrome, a condition that precedes the development of diabetes. It is about how to identify Metabolic Syndrome, how to avoid it and how to treat it. This book is about moderation. This book is about the changes in your lifestyle that will help you prevent the metabolic diseases and live a long, healthy, and productive life in this new era of medicine.

Adult-onset diabetes is increasingly seen *in children,* a devastating consequence of childhood obesity. Six million children in the US are obese.

Diabetes causes multiple life-threatening complications, including heart attacks, strokes, blindness, end stage kidney disease, amputations and nerve disease. The price tag to society from diabetes-related complications is staggering. Each year in the US, 160 billion dollars are spent on diabetes. The vast majority of diabetics have cardiovascular disease (CVD); most die from it.

Over the last 3 decades, substantial research has been done to explain the root causes and the interrelationships of obesity, diabetes and cardiovascular disease. It has been shown that these three conditions share a common underlying physiologic defect: *insulin resistance*.

In 1988, Dr Gerald Reaven defined Syndrome X, in which insulin resistance was shown to be the unifying abnormality for a cluster of risk factors for heart disease. These include an abnormal lipid panel (high triglycerides and low HDL), glucose intolerance, high blood pressure and high uric acid. With further research in large population groups, the concept of Syndrome X evolved into Metabolic Syndrome, a constellation of metabolic abnormalities (obesity, glucose intolerance, abnormal lipid pattern, high blood pressure) which predispose these individuals to coronary artery disease.

In 1998, the World Health Organization recognized the importance of Metabolic Syndrome as an important precursor to coronary artery disease and diabetes and proposed defining criteria for the syndrome. It was recognized that among patients with heart disease or diabetes, the majority have qualified as having Metabolic Syndrome for years preceding diagnosis. The underlying disorder in Metabolic Syndrome is insulin resistance—the other name for Metabolic Syndrome is Insulin Resistance Syndrome. In fact, this was the term used in the earlier draft of this book.

In general, the term diabetes implies that a patient does not produce enough insulin. This insulin deficiency could be relative or absolute. In the more common type of diabetes, the insulin deficiency is relative. The quantity of insulin is relatively OK, but the quality of its action is not. These people have *insulin resistance*. Being insulin resistant means the body does not respond to the effects of a given quantity of insulin the way a normal body should.

Insulin resistance in adult-onset diabetes has been known for a long time. What has been discovered more recently is the notion that insulin resistance can precede the onset of diabetes by several years, or even decades. These insulin-resistant people keep their blood sugar under control by producing more insulin than a normal person would, and in fact, they may have double the normal circulating level of insulin in the blood. The more insulin resistant the person is, the more insulin his/her pancreas must produce to control blood sugar. These elevated insulin levels, otherwise known as hyperinsulinemia, may be responsible for the majority of findings of Metabolic Syndrome.

Metabolic Syndrome is significant for a number of reasons. It plays a major role in the development of adult-onset diabetes, as well as coronary heart disease, independently from diabetes. All of the constituents of Metabolic Syndrome are well known risk factors for heart disease. Metabolic Syndrome leads to heart disease and heart attacks and should be treated as soon as it is diagnosed.

Despite advances in treatment and prevention, coronary artery disease (CAD) remains the single largest killer of men and women in the United States. Metabolic Syndrome is only now becoming generally recognized as a risk factor for CAD, despite overwhelming evidence in the scientific spheres. Knowing that you have the syndrome may prompt you to make daily changes in your life and prevent a life threatening disease.

Metabolic Syndrome may be easily identified. The typical patient is overweight, with the weight tending to be centered in the abdomen. Blood pressure is commonly borderline or elevated. The total cholesterol is often normal, but analysis of cholesterol subtypes reveals low HDL and high triglycerides. Blood sugar may be mildly elevated, but not high enough to be called diabetes. Many of these patients have a family member with diabetes. 25% or more of the adult population in the US show the signs of Metabolic Syndrome. Not all of them will develop diabetes or CAD, but until more is known, WHY TAKE CHANCES?

Treatment of Metabolic Syndrome is possible, through weight loss, exercise, dietary measures, and medications. As it turns out, weight loss and exercise each have an independent beneficial effect, meaning that you can benefit from exercise even if you are not able to shed weight. We also have a number of new medications that target the insulin resistance underlying Metabolic Syndrome.

What is the relationship of insulin resistance, diabetes, obesity and heart attacks? And why do they all happen to occur in the same people? A combination of environment and genetics acting together underlies most medical diseases. Obesity, insulin resistance, diabetes and coronary artery disease are all about this interaction of genes with environment. We cannot do much about the genes, but there is plenty of transformation that can and should be done to change our environment.

This book will outline what happens in the body during the decades before the development of diabetes and cardiovascular disease. We will discuss the pattern of findings (lipid profile, blood pressure, family history, body fat distribution and other signs) that together form the constellation of Metabolic Syndrome.

Where do you start?

- Learn about your family history, particularly regarding close relatives who have had diabetes (even at late age) and heart disease.

- Find out your cholesterol pattern.

- Weigh yourself and check your blood pressure regularly.

- Take a closer look at your lifestyle and diet.

- Make the changes in your lifestyle necessary to bring your weight into the ideal range.

- Stay current with developments in this exciting area of research.

This book is about all of the above. It is about Metabolic Syndrome, how to identify it, how to successfully treat it and, importantly, how to avoid its complications. This book is about moderation: think moderation, practice modification.

—Mariam Manoukian MD, PhD

OVERVIEW

*Tell them what you're going to say, say it,
then tell them what you've said.*

—old public speaking adage

You may be one of the 25 percent of people in the United States who are insulin resistant. Perhaps you've been told you show signs of insulin resistance. Even if you haven't been told, you may show signs such as pot-belly and high triglycerides, or maybe you have a family history of adult-onset diabetes, or maybe you've had some success with a high-protein, low carbohydrate diet.

The concept of insulin resistance is that your pancreas (insulin-secreting gland) needs to produce more insulin than normal to control your blood sugar when you eat carbohydrates (sugar or starch). You can think of it as if your pancreas is shouting at your body (by producing more insulin) because your body isn't paying attention. We tend to compare it with yelling at our children when they don't pay attention to us.

Are we yelling at our children because they are ignoring us? Or are they ignoring us because we are yelling at them? Is your pancreas producing so much insulin because your body is resistant to insulin's effects? Or is your body resistant to the effects because it has been flooded with so much insulin?

Many insulin-resistant people develop diabetes during their lifetime. While diabetes can cause many problems, including damage to eyes, feet, etc., its major health effect is that it leads to cardiovascular disease. Most diabetics develop coronary artery disease and are at risk for heart attacks. (Half of adult-onset diabetics already have coronary disease by the time they are diagnosed with diabetes!) It has been shown, however, that the increased risk of coronary disease is not simply in the diabetic few, but *in all insulin-resistant people.* Treating insulin resistance is, therefore, a major goal in the prevention of heart disease and stroke.

Measuring insulin resistance (or insulin sensitivity) can be done precisely in a clinical laboratory using methods that are not appropriate for day-to-day use. However, by recognizing the characteristic features of the Metabolic Syndrome, we can quite easily diagnose insulin resistance. These features include borderline (or high) blood sugar, fat distribution centered around the waist or "pot belly," high blood pressure, high triglycerides, and low levels of the protective HDL cholesterol. Sometimes there is high uric acid or history of gout.

Think of it like this. If we, the physicians, labeled all of our patients as insulin resistant, we would be correct at least 20–25 percent of the time. This is because 25% of the general population *is* insulin resistant. Now if we were a bit more selective, for instance diagnosing everyone with a pot belly as being insulin resistant and having Metabolic Syndrome, our accuracy would increase, possibly to 70-80 percent. Imagine now, that we can further refine our accuracy by knowing that a patient's blood pressure is high, or that he/she suffers from gout, or that there is a family history of diabetes. Consider that we can measure laboratory parameters such as blood sugar, uric acid and cholesterol profile. Insulin resistance as part of Metabolic Syndrome becomes easier to diagnose than a common cold!

Treatment of Metabolic Syndrome is not quite so easy as its diagnosis. After all, it requires a change in our behavior. Specific recommendations can be made, and these involve exercise, weight loss, and carbohydrate restriction. We have tried to make this as painless as possible.

—Jerry Manoukian, MD

PART I

The Footprints of Metabolic Syndrome

METABOLIC SYNDROME is characterized by insulin resistance, abdominal weight gain, characteristic pattern of lipid profile, glucose intolerance and high blood pressure. Other features of Metabolic Syndrome include tendency to blood clotting and gout. The correlation of obesity and insulin resistance is similar to the chicken and egg. If you are obese, particularly around the stomach, you are insulin resistant. If you are insulin resistant, then you are gaining weight around the stomach and have a hard time losing it.

The purpose of insulin is to help our bodies control the use of sugar in the blood for fuel. Secreted from the pancreas, insulin maintains a stable level of glucose in the blood, and keeps it from going up too high when we eat sugar or starch. Thanks to these flexible levels of insulin, in healthy individuals the blood glucose never rises above 140–150 mg/dl. If you have genes that predispose you to insulin resistance, the insulin action becomes less effective with time and harder work is required from the pancreas to keep the glucose level from climbing over the border into the diabetic range (hyperglycemia). Many patients are found to have both high glucose in the blood (hyperglycemia) and higher than normal insulin production (hyperinsulinemia). These high levels of insulin are needed because the person is less sensitive to insulin's signal in the cells. Insulin sensitivity is the opposite of insulin resistance: the more insulin resistant a person is, the less sensitive he is. As an analogy, the taller you are, the less short you are. Your eventual height is predetermined by heredity, with some contribution from your environment.

Who are the people with genetic predisposition to Metabolic Syndrome? These are people who have a relative with Type 2 or adult-onset diabetes, women who have polycystic ovary syndrome, women who have had gestational diabetes, and the aging population in general. Certain ethnic groups, including Hispanics, African-Americans, Asian Indians, and Native Americans are at high risk. These are people who are known to be at a risk for developing diabetes. Once insulin resistance genes and obesity with sedentary lifestyle have found each other, Metabolic Syndrome develops.

What is the culprit in the development of insulin resistance? There are many theories. The current notion is that increased free fatty acid levels in the blood play a major role. Most of the free fatty acids (FFA) in the blood stream come from the breakdown of body fat, so-called adipose tissue. Elevated levels of FFA act on the liver, which is an important action site for insulin, causing insulin resistance. FFA also cause muscle tissue to become more insulin resistant, impairing the uptake of glucose by muscles, which have become less sensitive to insulin's signals. Increased entry of FFA into the liver is also responsible for the typical pattern of dyslipidemia with increased triglycerides and low HDL.

When healthy individuals are given an intravenous infusion of FFA, they show an instant decrease in insulin sensitivity. People with increased fat in the abdominal area (Apple shape) will flood the liver with FFA as they break down their intraabdominal fat. The released FFA will get a shortcut into the liver and create obstacles for insulin action, causing insulin resistance.

Fat that lies within the abdominal cavity shares the same blood supply as the intestines. Veins draining the abdominal cavity don't drain blood directly to the heart in the same way that the veins drain blood from other parts of the body. Instead, they drain through the portal vein to the liver. In this way, the sandwich you had for lunch will be detoxified by the liver before flowing back to the rest of the body. When abdominal fat is used between the meals, the released FFA will drain to the liver. The liver becomes more insulin resistant on this high fat diet.

Where there is insulin resistance, there is hyperinsulinemia. These two entities go hand-in-hand. Elevated insulin levels develop to maintain the stable level of blood glucose. This is a hard job for the pancreas, as it has to work to come up with more and more insulin. For years, balance is maintained as high insulin levels keep the blood sugar in normal range. When fasting sugar is checked during a routine exam, it is normal and the person is reassured in his good health. In the meantime, insulin resistance and hyperinsulinemia are causing or underlying several metabolic abnormalities, including an abnormal cholesterol profile, high blood pressure, easy blood clotting (hypercoagulability), and high uric acid levels (the cause of gout). The person is now at high risk for a heart attack.

In *The Little Prince* by Antoine De Saint Exupery, the little boy draws a picture looking like this.

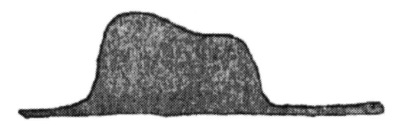

SOURCE: *The Little Prince* by Antoine De Saint-Exupery. Harcourt Trade Publishers (with permission).

Then he asks the grown-ups whether the drawing frightens them. They answer, "Frightened? Why should a hat frighten anyone?" Well, the drawing is not a hat. It is a picture of a boa constrictor digesting an elephant.

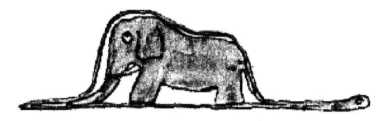

Source: *The Little Prince* by Antoine De Saint-Exupery. Harcourt Trade Publishers (with permission).

Analogy can be made for Metabolic Syndrome. For years, people with Metabolic Syndrome are thought to be healthy. However, they have been harboring metabolic abnormalities, perhaps not enough to be called a disease, but quite enough to make them high risk for a heart attack. Frequently, diabetes is diagnosed during the first heart attack. Why? How? Because the person had Metabolic Syndrome for years and the clock for CAD started to tick long before the onset of diabetes. Because in this population, CAD and diabetes have the same root cause—the insulin resistance and hyperinsulinemia.

Most people with obesity have some degree of insulin resistance. Not all of them will show the features of Metabolic Syndrome. Only people with genetic predisposition have Metabolic Syndrome. These tend to be individuals with the preferential distribution of fat around their waist and the characteristic lipid panel. They may have close family members with diabetes, again suggesting the importance of genes.

In 1988, Dr Gerald Reaven from Stanford described Syndrome X as a cluster of metabolic abnormalities including adult onset diabetes or impaired glucose tolerance, abnormal cholesterol profile (high triglycerides, low HDL), high blood pressure (hypertension), and their association with high insulin levels (hyperinsulinemia). Subsequently, other conditions were noted to belong to this syndrome, including increased clotting, decreased ability to dissolve clots, and slow clearance of fat from the bloodstream following a meal. All these conditions are known promoters of heart disease. Other names were tried for the syndrome, such as "Insulin Resistance Syndrome," "plurimetabolic syndrome," "dysmetabolic syndrome X," "cardiovascular syndrome," or "deadly quartet." The terms Insulin Resistance Syndrome and Metabolic Syndrome are often used interchangeably, but since Metabolic Syndrome is the term accepted worldwide, that is the name we use in this book.

Now we're going to make an important point. Dr Reaven made his discovery by directly measuring the insulin sensitivity of his subjects, a very labor-intense process. In large population studies, researchers made their conclusions based on measurement of insulin levels in the blood. In office practice, neither of these approaches is done routinely. *Thus, the diagnosis of insulin resistance must be based on the associated findings, the so-called "Footprints of Metabolic Syndrome."*

The definitions of Metabolic Syndrome vary slightly between the National Cholesterol Education Program and WHO guidelines, but there is a great deal of overlap (*see* Tables 1 and 2).

TABLE 1

Guidelines for Clinical Identification of Metabolic Syndrome (NCEP ATP III)*

Presence of 3 or more of these risk factors qualifies patient for Metabolic Syndrome.

Risk factor	Defining level
Abdominal obesity (waist circumference)	Waist circumference
Men	>40 in
Women	>35 in
Triglycerides	>150 mg/dl
High density cholesterol (HDL)	
Men	<40 mg/dl
Women	<50 mg/dl
Blood pressure	>130/85 mm Hg
Fasting glucose	>110 mg/dl

*Source: National Cholesterol Education Program Adult Treatment Panel III, *JAMA* (2001), 285:2486-2497

TABLE 2

World Health Organization (WHO) Definition of Metabolic Syndrome

Glucose abnormality demonstrated by
- Type 2 diabetes or impaired fasting glucose *or*
- Impaired glucose tolerance and/or insulin resistance
- *Plus* 2 or more of the following risk factors

Risk factor	Defining level
Waist:hip ratio	>0.9 for men and >0.85 for women
Triglycerides	>150
or HDL	<35 for men and <45 for women
Blood pressure	>160/90
Microalbuminuria	> 20 mcg/min

Impaired fasting glucose is defined as a fasting glucose level between 110 and 125 (original WHO definition).

Impaired glucose tolerance is defined as abnormally high blood sugar (>140 mg/dl) in response to a standard glucose drink.

Insulin resistance is defined as a high insulin level above the 75th percentile or decreased insulin action as measured in a specialized laboratory.

Source: *Diabetes Medicine* (1998). 15:539-553.

There is plenty of evidence that the syndrome exists in the population and is associated with coronary artery disease. Compared with non-insulin resistant people, those with higher levels of insulin have twice as much chance of developing hypertension, three times as much chance of developing the characteristic cholesterol patterns, and 6 times more chance of developing diabetes. All these are risk factors for CAD, with heart attack being the ultimate result if untreated. Using the NCEP ATP III guidelines, national survey data suggest roughly 25% of US adults over 20 years of age are affected by Metabolic Syndrome. The incidence dramatically increases with age, from 7% among people in their 20s to over 40% for people over age 60. The syndrome is more common in Mexican Americans (women 36%, men 28%). The prevalence of Metabolic

Syndrome will increase as populations age and become more obese. White women (23%) and white men (25%) in the US are equally affected. Overall, 24% of white persons, 22% of African Americans, and 32% of Mexican Americans in the US are affected. Using the NCEP ATP III criteria, one study in the United States showed that 83% of diabetics had Metabolic Syndrome. A study done in Canada showed that 51% of patients with coronary artery disease had Metabolic Syndrome.

The figure shown below outlines the relationship between heredity, lifestyle, Metabolic Syndrome, its associated findings, and development of diabetes and CAD. Glucose intolerance is shown as a prediabetic state, when the blood sugar is elevated after meals, but is not yet to the point that it is called diabetes.

Components of the Metabolic Syndrome

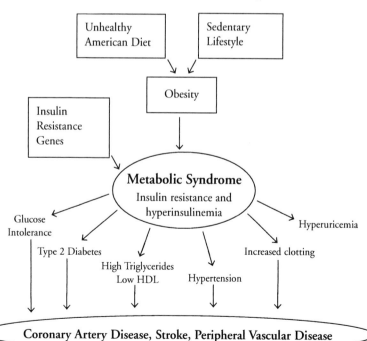

We'll briefly discuss each one of the components of Metabolic Syndrome. Because increased clotting is not measurable by routine testing, it is not formally part of Metabolic Syndrome; it is, however, one of the features that makes Metabolic Syndrome so dangerous.

Insulin resistance and Metabolic Syndrome are associated with a defect in the body's ability to dissolve clots when they form, a process known as fibrinolysis. This may have serious consequences, such as when a clot forms over the surface of a cholesterol plaque in a coronary artery. If the body is unable to dissolve the clot in time, it may block the vessel and cause a heart attack.

Plasminogen activator inhibitor 1 (PAI-1, pronounced "pie-one") is produced by the body as an inhibitor of fibrinolysis, and counteracts the body's efforts to dissolve clots once they form. Elevated levels of PAI-1 have been found in patients with coronary artery disease, hypertension, obesity, hypertriglyceridemia, and diabetes, all conditions associated with hyperinsulinemia and insulin resistance.

High levels of uric acid in the blood can lead to gout and certain types of urinary stones. It is associated with Metabolic Syndrome, but is not felt to be a risk factor for coronary artery disease. PAI-1 and uric acid are not defining criteria for Metabolic Syndrome. PAI-1 is too difficult to measure, and uric acid's importance in Metabolic Syndrome is not completely understood.

1

Obesity

Obese: [from Latin, obedere, to eat away]

Metabolic Syndrome is very common, affecting 25-30% of the population. Remember, we said that if we labeled all of our patients as being insulin resistant, we'd be correct at least 25 percent of the time. Most insulin-resistant people are overweight. Conversely, virtually all obese people are insulin resistant, to some degree.

What is the Definition of Obesity?

The definition of obesity offered by World Health Organization (WHO) is based on the measurement of body mass index (BMI). Your BMI is your weight in kilograms divided by the square of your height in meters. BMI = weight (kg)/height (m^2). Obesity is defined as BMI >30 kg/m^2. BMI >25 kg/m^2 is considered overweight. There are charts that you can use to identify your BMI, as well as to see exactly what your weight should or should not be. The ideal BMI is probably 19–23 kg/m^2 for women and 20–24 kg/m^2 for men. If you are a larger frame person, then up to 25 kg/m^2 is OK. We have included a BMI chart with dimensions given in pounds and inches (*see* Table 3).

TABLE 3

Find Your Body Mass Index (BMI)

Height (inches)

Weight (lbs.)	58	59	60	61	62	63	64	65	66	67	68	69	70	71	72	73	74	75	76
100	21	20	20	19	18	18	17	17	16	16	15	15	14	14	14	13	13	12	12
105	22	21	21	20	19	19	18	17	17	16	16	16	15	15	14	14	13	13	13
110	23	22	21	21	20	19	19	18	18	17	17	16	16	15	15	15	14	14	13
115	24	23	22	22	21	20	20	19	19	18	17	17	17	16	16	15	15	14	14
120	25	24	23	23	22	21	21	20	19	19	18	18	17	17	16	16	15	15	15
125	26	25	24	24	23	22	21	21	20	20	19	18	18	17	17	16	16	16	15
130	27	26	25	25	24	23	22	22	21	20	20	19	19	18	18	17	17	16	16
135	28	27	26	26	25	24	23	22	22	21	21	20	19	19	18	18	17	17	16
140	29	28	27	26	26	25	24	23	23	22	21	21	20	20	19	18	18	17	17
145	30	29	28	27	27	26	25	24	23	23	22	21	21	20	20	19	19	18	18
150	31	30	29	28	27	27	26	25	24	23	23	22	22	21	20	20	19	19	18
155	32	31	30	29	28	27	27	26	25	24	24	23	22	22	21	20	20	19	19
160	33	32	31	30	29	28	27	27	26	25	24	24	23	22	22	21	21	20	19
165	34	33	32	31	30	29	28	27	27	26	25	24	24	23	22	22	21	21	20
170	35	34	33	32	31	30	29	28	27	27	26	25	24	24	23	22	22	21	21
175	36	35	34	33	32	31	30	29	28	27	27	26	25	24	24	23	22	22	21
180	37	36	35	34	33	32	31	30	29	28	27	27	26	25	24	24	23	22	22
185	39	37	36	35	34	33	32	31	30	29	28	27	27	26	25	24	24	23	23
190	40	38	37	36	35	34	33	32	31	30	29	28	27	26	26	25	24	24	23
195	41	39	38	37	36	35	33	32	31	31	30	29	28	27	26	26	25	24	24
200	42	40	39	38	37	35	34	33	32	31	30	30	29	28	27	26	26	25	24
205	43	41	40	39	37	36	35	34	33	32	31	30	29	29	28	27	26	26	25
210	44	42	41	40	38	37	36	35	34	33	32	31	30	29	28	28	27	26	26
215	45	43	42	41	39	38	37	36	35	34	33	32	31	30	29	28	28	27	26
220	46	44	43	42	40	39	38	37	36	34	33	32	32	31	30	29	28	27	27
225	47	45	44	43	41	40	39	37	36	35	34	33	32	31	31	30	29	28	27
230	48	46	45	43	42	41	39	38	37	36	35	34	33	32	31	30	30	29	28
235	49	47	46	44	43	42	40	39	38	37	36	35	34	33	32	31	30	29	29

Look up your BMI from the chart, circle it on the graph, and write it in the box below. If your BMI is below 23 kg/m^2, you may skip this chapter, unless you tend to gain weight around your waist.

My BMI is

Now follow the graph up from your circled BMI number until you see the first box with a 25 or 26 in it. From this, you can see the weight at which you have a normal BMI.

For a BMI of 25, my weight should be

Are You an Apple or a Pear?

People gain weight with different patterns. Some (men or women) gain more weight around the waist, which is the "male pattern." This type of obesity, looking like an apple, is called abdominal, android or central type. Another weight gain pattern (men or women) is excessive weight around the buttocks, the "female pattern." This type of obesity is called a gynoid type or general obesity, and the body shape resembles a pear.

All people who are obese are, to some degree, insulin resistant. However, people with abdominal obesity are far more insulin resistant. Why? One hypothesis is that the fat tissue from the

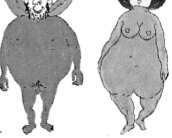

ANDROID TYPE   GYNOID TYPE

abdominal region is more metabolically relevant. Abdominal fat is in closer proximity to the liver than is subcutaneous fat; therefore, it releases free fatty acids that directly drain into the liver (through a special system called the portal veins) and create obstacles for insulin action. When the abdominal fat was measured with a special technique called DEXA scan in both obese and lean individuals, it was the intra-abdominal fat that showed stronger correlation with insulin resistance than did the overall obesity. Abdominal obesity strongly correlates with high blood pressure, coronary artery disease and tendency for clotting. It is likely that the common denominator for these effects is insulin resistance. Abdominal obesity and insulin resistance have a dual relationship. Abdominal obesity stimulates insulin resistance—insulin resistance promotes weight gain. The more you eat, the more insulin is produced. But because of insulin resistance, the fat cell senses insulin *deficiency* and determines that it is time to eat.

Even if your BMI is below 25 kg/m^2, you still might be insulin resistant. One limitation of BMI is that it does not distinguish between the two different patterns of obesity. Another measure can be used for that purpose: the Waist-to-Hip ratio (ratio of waist circumference to hip girth). A ratio of 0.85 and more is characteristic for abdominal obesity. The simplest way to determine your pattern is to look in the mirror. If you have a large belly, not much buttocks and thin extremities, you are likely to be an apple.

Here's a short real life story.

Years ago when we had to work too many hours, we had two babysitters, Anna and Hanna, for our daughter. They were similar age, both in their late fifties, and both were moderately obese; both were relatively healthy, not taking any medications at the time. The difference in these ladies was the distribution of their weight. Anna had a large belly and thin legs and arms, looking just like a classical *apple*. Hanna's weight was mostly around her buttocks, arms and legs, with a less pronounced belly, looking like a *pear*. Six years later, Anna was diagnosed with diabetes, high blood pressure and dyslipidemia and was taking multiple medications; Hanna was mostly struggling with pains and aches in her knees.

Why is it "Bad" to be Obese?

Ample studies have shown that people with obesity have an increased tendency toward developing diabetes, high blood pressure, dyslipidemia and cardiovascular diseases, and that they live shorter lives than lean people. There is a correlation between the BMI and risk for diabetes, with one study showing that being overweight at the age 25 is a strong predictor of diabetes in middle age. Another study showed that middle-age men who gained more than 10% of their weight after age 20 were significantly more likely to have Metabolic Syndrome. However, not all overweight or obese people are going to have diabetes or heart attack—those who have Metabolic Syndrome will most likely suffer from these complications.

What are the Causes of Obesity?

Obesity is a multifactorial disease involving interactions among genetic, endocrine, metabolic, environmental and cultural factors. Studies of obese individuals and their relatives, identical and fraternal twins, and even identical twins raised apart suggest that the genetic contribution to obesity is 40–65%. Genes are very important. The saying "You are what you eat," is not entirely true. "You are what your genes are," is a more fair statement. Still, about $^1/_3$ of obesity is caused by the environment, especially the foods you eat and a sedentary lifestyle.

Leptin is a hormone secreted by fat cells and is thought to cause satiety, the feeling of having eaten enough. Circulating leptin concentrations are highly correlated with the level of obesity. Administration of leptin to animals leads to acute decrease in food intake. It is clear that the brain is an important site of leptin action. Severe obesity is described in people who have resistance to leptin, though it is shown to be a rare condition. This is all very new research and needs more investigation.

Another hormone, ghrelin, is a powerful appetite-stimulating hormone and has been found in very high concentrations in the central nervous systems of obese individuals. It was discovered very recently and is receiving significant attention.

Metabolism is often slowed down in obesity. The energy intake outbalances the energy expenditure and excess energy is accumulated as fat. People with obesity gain weight easily and have a harder time losing it when compared to the lean individuals. When compared to people without diabetes, individuals with diabetes and obesity have a harder time losing weight.

Environmental factors are extremely important. The food supply and variety is growing, particularly fast food and sugared beverages, while at the same time, physical activity is declining. If somebody consumes a high fat, high Calorie diet and entertains himself watching TV for hours while lying on the couch, then no wonder the result is weight gain of 10–30 pounds per year. There is correlation between the number of hours spent watching TV per week and level of obesity in children, as well as correlation between obesity and number of TVs in the household. Don't be surprised if a similar correlation is found between obesity and hours spent with computer games.

Cultural factors are also very important. Personal attitudes toward body weight and fatness vary among different social and cultural groups, with these differences in attitude undoubtedly affecting rates of obesity. In some countries, obesity is a symbol of affluence, and thus is to be desired. High prevalence of obesity among older African-American and Hispanic women appears to be more acceptable, perhaps a symbol of motherhood and dignity. In contrast, in the US and Western Europe, affluent people usually shun obesity. Social pressure mounts against obesity in adolescence, causing different eating disorders in this age group.

Another cause of overeating and obesity is the stress of adult life. Too much competition and challenge compound the usual stresses of social and family responsibilities, and a common response to stress is to fall back on pleasurable escapes (chocolate, chips, and cheese puffs). Frequently, people admit going to the refrigerator to relieve nervous tension.

How Do We Gain Weight?

Imagine a large balance scale with a genetic predisposition at the base. The left dish has the energy intake: a high-Calorie, high-fat diet; the right dish has the energy expenditure, including exercise. It is all simple arithmetic. If your energy intake is more than your expenditure, you will gain weight.

Energy comes in the form of food and is used for basal metabolic needs and physical activity. Surplus is stored as fat.

Total Calories = Metabolic needs + physical exercise + fat storage
(food)   (weight gain)

or

Fat storage = (food intake) − (metabolic needs + exercise)

In other words, energy can neither be created nor destroyed; it is just transformed from one form to another.

This extra intake can happen subtly. If you eat as few as 100 extra Calories every day for one year, you will gain 12 pounds in 1 year. A 4-ounce non-fat frozen yogurt, 1 apple or 2 tablespoons of sunflower seeds, each of these is equal to 100 Calories. Things like these are usually eaten without counting or paying attention.

Why is the Prevalence of Obesity Increasing in the US?

An epidemic of obesity in the US is frequently being reported in the news. Childhood obesity is a growing problem. In 1962, 43% of the population in the US was overweight or obese; in 1994 that number reached 55%. In 2002 it was around 60%. Approximately 100 million Americans, almost 3 out of 5 adults, are overweight or obese. This is not because of changing genetics; genes just don't change this quickly. While some major risk factors, like cigarette smoking, have started to decline, and high blood pressure and cholesterol levels are better treated than ever before, obesity and diabetes are on the rise.

Much of this starts from childhood. Sedentary lifestyle and increased portions of high fat, high carbohydrate meals are responsible for growing obesity. Let us look at some everyday culprits of this problem.

- Fast food chains serving high fat, high carbohydrate meals that are enjoyed universally. Working moms are saved from prolonged traditional cooking; there are no dirty dishes and kids love it.

- Lots of snacks that are high in fat and carbohydrates and low in fiber. Many companies fill up the break rooms with candy, chips, sodas, and chocolate chip cookies. It tastes even better when it is free.

- Traditional American parties with chips and dips, burgers and hot dogs, piñatas and party bags filled with candy. Not to mention "trick or treat."

- Personal cars for everybody, escalators, elevators.

- Computers, videos, video games.

All these factors have a history of accepted behaviors for several decades, resulting in the epidemic of obesity. The rising incidence of Type 2 diabetes is due to increasing obesity and sedentary lifestyle, both of which promote insulin resistance.

Treatment of Obesity

Treatment of obesity is the same as treatment of Metabolic Syndrome: a lifestyle change with a proper diet and exercise. These are discussed in later chapters.

Here, we will review available *prescription* medications and surgical options for severe obesity. Drug treatment of obesity has not been very successful for several reasons. Obesity is a chronic disease, just like hypertension and diabetes, and its treatment should be lifelong. Primary treatment of obesity is lifestyle change that also should be lifelong. The common scenario is this: the patient asks for a "jump start," then loses some weight, is satisfied and slowly slides back into the previous lifestyle, regaining the weight. This is why we continue to emphasize LIFESTYLE change, yours and everybody else's around you.

Regarding medications: for the last 30–40 years, many different anti-obesity drugs and supplements appeared and then were dropped from the market. Whenever used, pros and cons of these medications should be discussed with your doctor. Currently there are three different types of medications on the market. Two of those are appetite suppressors and work in the brain. The third inhibits fat absorption. They all have similar benefit, which is an average weight loss of 5–10% of the starting weight in the 50–60% of patients who respond to treatment. With this seemingly modest level of weight loss, there is an improvement of the risk profile *if* the weight is maintained. We remind you that all the medications work only *if* they are supported by the diet.

Phentermine is a generic drug (appetite suppressor) that has been on the market since the 1960s. It is chemically related to amphetamines and has a potential for addiction. It is approved for short-term use only. It may cause nervousness, shakiness and headache. It was part of Fen-Phen treatment that helped many patients lose weight, but was later linked to heart valve damage.

Sibutramine (Meridia) is another appetite suppressant with a different mechanism of action. It has been on the market for a little more than 3 years. It is contraindicated in the patients with uncontrolled blood pressure. Headache, racing heart, insomnia and nervousness are the main side effects that occur in about 20% of patients.

Orlistat (Xenical) is another new drug that works by blocking 30% of the total fat intake when the medication is taken with meals. In order to be absorbed, fat from the meal first is broken down into smaller subunits and then penetrates into the intestinal wall. Xenical blocks the enzyme that helps absorb the fat and it is excreted with the stool. Main side effects include gastrointestinal symptoms, such as greasy stools and stool incontinence. The side effects commonly occur if the meal was high in fat content. If you are on this medication and are having too many side effects, your diet probably contains too much fat.

So far, not much to brag about. Studies with leptin (the appetite suppressive hormone) in animals have been promising, but nothing is yet known for humans. Appetite and hunger are complex functions based on interactions between the brain and the digestive tract and societal stimuli. To interrupt this complex puzzle with a pill is an ambitious undertaking, indeed. Further, the heart valve issues resulting from the Fen-Phen combination demonstrate how dangerous side effects can be.

Weight loss surgery (bariatric surgery) is a mechanical form of treatment. The stomach is usually stapled or bypassed, so there is no room to store food. Appetite diminishes because of nausea and a feeling of fullness. Surgery had been restricted to very obese people (BMI greater than 40, or BMI greater than 35 *plus* complications from obesity). The most common surgery is the gastric bypass, otherwise known as Roux-en-Y surgery. A small pouch is made out of the stomach and is connected to the part of the intestine called the jejunum. A large part of the stomach and the duodenum, where most of the food is absorbed, is removed from the gastrointestinal tract. After this surgery, people have less appetite and most of the eaten food is not absorbed. Another procedure (a band around the stomach that is done without major surgery) is now approved for weight loss. It has not been very successful and is not done as commonly as gastric bypass. A new procedure under investigation involves a small device similar to a pacemaker. It is implanted under the skin with an electrode implanted in the stomach, causing a sensation of fullness. Even though these procedures sound like extreme measures, they may be appropriate for severely obese people.

In summary, obesity is a chronic disease and needs a lifelong commitment. For an obese person, even a 5–7% weight loss per year can make a difference and will improve the metabolic abnormalities and insulin resistance. Prevention of the obesity is an even more important and rewarding job. Teach your children about obesity, teach them healthy habits, a healthy lifestyle, be your own doctor and your children's doctor, and you will prevent obesity, diabetes, heart disease and much more.

2

Diabetes

Traditionally, people assume that diabetes is a disease of elevated blood sugar and not enough insulin. This is both true and not true. It all depends on what type of diabetes we are talking about.

Types of Diabetes

There are several types of diabetes. Type 1 and Type 2 are the common ones. Juvenile onset (Type 1 or insulin-dependent diabetes) is the one that occurs commonly in young, thin individuals. It is caused by damage to the pancreas by the patient's own immune system. From the beginning of the illness, the pancreas is unable to produce insulin and patients require lifelong insulin injections to sustain normal body functions. Type 1 diabetes is not addressed in this book.

Adult onset, also known as Type 2 or non-insulin dependent diabetes, is the most common type of diabetes. More than 90% of diabetics have this type of diabetes, and in this book we refer to it as adult-onset diabetes mellitus or simply diabetes; it generally occurs in older people (over age 40). Recently, with the epidemic of obesity, the age of onset of Type 2 diabetes is decreasing; it is starting to affect younger people. Adult onset diabetes is more and more seen in children, solely because of childhood obesity. If Type 1 diabetes is characterized by *absolute* insulin deficiency, Type 2 diabetes is characterized by insulin resistance and *relative* insulin deficiency. In adult-onset diabetes, the pancreas makes some (or a lot of) insulin, but it is still not enough to keep the blood sugar within normal limits because of the patient's insulin resistance. The majority of patients that we see in the office have Type 2 diabetes.

Relationship of Metabolic Syndrome and Diabetes

Metabolic Syndrome is a prediabetic state. Although an estimated 25% of the population is insulin resistant, only about 6% to 15% of the population becomes diabetic. Who are these people? Again, it is about genes. People with a genetic predisposition to diabetes develop a failure in insulin secretion, and the blood sugar level rises. These people progress from Metabolic Syndrome with normal glucose tolerance, to impaired glucose tolerance, and subsequently to diabetes.

An early defect in the insulin-secreting pattern has been found in patients with Metabolic Syndrome prone to developing diabetes. The insulin secreting cells fail because of the genetic defect in the insulin-secreting cells of the pancreas. In the future, genetic testing may help to identify these patients years before they develop diabetes.

Impaired Fasting Glucose and Impaired Glucose Tolerance

Two important terms to understand are impaired fasting glucose (IFG) and impaired glucose tolerance (IGT). Both of these conditions are defining criteria of Metabolic Syndrome. In both conditions, there is enough insulin to prevent blood sugar from rising above the levels called "diabetic," but not enough insulin to keep the blood sugar truly "normal." Recall that there may still be more insulin present in these individuals than in a truly normal person, but that the action of insulin is hampered by the body's insulin resistance.

IFG is a fasting blood sugar of 100–125 mg/dl. This is less than the cutoff of 126 mg/dl required to diagnose diabetes, but is above the truly normal fasting level of 80–100 mg/dl. In November 2003, the lower cutoff level for IFG was changed from 110 mg/dl to 100 mg/dl, because these lower numbers were recognized as predictive of diabetes later in life.

IGT refers to the blood sugar rise after a meal. During a standard test, the patient drinks a solution containing 75 grams of glucose. If the blood sugar rises to between 140 and 200 mg/dl during the next two hours, the patient is said to have IGT. Note that we don't call the patient diabetic unless the blood sugar rises above 200 mg/dl at two hours. Five percent of these glucose intolerant individuals will progress to overt diabetes *per year.* The significance of IFG and IGT is that both of these conditions are prediabetic states. Both conditions are characteristic of Metabolic Syndrome and both are associated with increased rates of CAD. Without aggressive intervention, they will progress to diabetes.

How Does Diabetes Develop?

Diabetes is a disease of metabolism involving many organ systems. It is a disease of pancreas, muscle, liver and fat tissue. Glucose level is only a marker of the disease, the tip of the iceberg.

Normally, when glucose is absorbed from the intestine, its level increases in the blood. The pancreas secretes some additional insulin in response to that glucose, delivering it to the muscles and liver, keeping the "after meals" glucose level below 140–150 mg/dl. Muscle tissue uses the glucose for its own purposes, burning some for energy and storing the excess as glycogen. The liver uses glucose for its purposes, including storage as glycogen. When we are fasting (several hours since the last meal), stored glucose is released into the blood to maintain glucose in the blood at a certain level (above 80 mg/dl and below 100 mg/dl).

Recall that under normal conditions, insulin produced by the pancreas (in response to high blood sugar) clears the blood of excess sugar. It does so by opening the way for glucose to travel into the muscles and the liver. Special receptors in the muscles, liver and other tissues recognize the insulin and open the doors for glucose to enter. Because of insulin resistance, the insulin is unable to create the desired lowering of blood sugar. The pancreas compensates by producing more insulin (hyperinsulinemia). This floods the body with insulin, and, hopefully, stimulates these receptors and lowers the blood sugar into the normal range.

When the pancreatic cells that produce insulin start to wear out, the pancreas is not able to maintain high levels of insulin needed to control blood sugar. What causes the insulin producing cells (beta cells) in the pancreas to wear out? It appears that there are multiple causes of beta cell failure and death, leading to failure of the pancreas to keep up with insulin production. This is believed to be the pivotal event leading to development of diabetes. High glucose levels in the blood are directly toxic to beta cells; high levels of free fatty acids (derived from breakdown of fat stores) are also toxic to beta cells. As you will recall from earlier, these free fatty acids also worsen insulin resistance, particularly in muscle and liver tissue.

Scientists still argue over what is the initial or primary problem in the development of diabetes: is it insulin resistance or insulin deficiency? Which is the chicken and which is the egg? Some researchers followed healthy relatives of diabetics for many years; they found out that insulin resistance at the beginning of the study was the main determinant of developing diabetes 20 years later. Others showed that years before the development of diabetes, the pattern of insulin secretion is changed (the early surge of insulin at the start of a meal is diminished), and the insulin resistance brought by obesity will unveil the disease.

Manifestations of Diabetes

Hyperglycemia (high glucose levels in the bloodstream) occurs because the body is less efficient at moving glucose into the organs that use it (i.e., liver, muscle and fat tissue). As blood is filtered through the kidneys, sugar spills into the urine, taking extra water with it. The presenting symptoms of the disease are frequent urination, thirst, and weight loss or weight gain, dry skin, blurry vision, and chronic tiredness. Bear in mind, however, that many diabetics have *no* symptoms! Therefore, screening of asymptomatic people for diabetes is an extremely important health policy.

Unfortunately, the natural progression of adult onset diabetes is a progressive failure of insulin secretion by the pancreas. With years of diabetes, the relative insulin insufficiency becomes more prominent and some people will eventually require insulin.

Within the last decade or so, the prevalence of cardiovascular disease is declining, but the number of people with diabetes and heart disease is growing, particularly among women. The good news is that we have a larger variety of, and more potent, medications than 5 years ago, and there are ways of preserving the pancreas.

Complications of Diabetes

Diabetes exerts many of its damaging effects on various organs by its effect on the blood vessels feeding these organs. Organs such as the heart, brain and limbs are affected by atherosclerotic blockage of the large blood vessels feeding them. Organs such as the kidneys, eyes and nerves are affected by diabetic damage to their microscopically small blood vessels.

Injury to small vessels has a different cause than atherosclerotic damage to the large blood vessels. Evidence shows that high blood sugar levels seen in diabetes directly harm small blood vessels. This may occur through the action of chemicals known as advanced glycation endproducts (AGEs). However, discussion of AGEs is beyond the scope of this book. You will likely hear about them in the years to come.

Often there is a mixed picture. While the brain is fed by large blood vessels, it is made of nerve tissue, which is fed by small vessels. Similarly, the kidneys can suffer small vessel damage to their delicate filtering structures, or shut down completely when the large arteries feeding them are blocked by cholesterol plaque. Foot ulcers are also a result of small vessel disease that damages the nerves to the feet, as well as blockage of large arteries feeding the legs.

Diabetes and Coronary Artery Disease (CAD)

Coronary artery disease (CAD) is the cause of angina and heart attacks. It remains the number one killer of Americans, accounting for over half the deaths in the US. Put in perspective, this translates to more deaths from CAD than from all other causes combined. The process is accelerated in diabetes, a leading cause of CAD. 80% of diabetics will die from the large-vessel complications (heart attack or stroke) if they are not aggressively prevented. Also, diabetics tend to suffer heart attacks and stroke at a lower age than non-diabetics.

Women without diabetes rarely suffer heart attacks before menopause because the female hormones provide protection from CAD. With diabetes, however, women lose that important hormonal benefit. Women with diabetes have no less risk than men of dying of a heart attack.

One of strongest predictors of a heart attack is that the patient has already had a previous heart attack. People who have had one heart attack have a dramatically higher risk of having another, when compared to people who have never had a heart attack. Diabetics have a risk of heart attack that is as high as for nondiabetics who have already had a heart attack. Thus, having diabetes carries an equivalent risk to having known CAD.

Are all these deaths caused solely by high blood sugar? Definitely not! Much, if not most, of the dirty work is done by high blood pressure, obesity, dyslipidemia, and prothrombotic state (tendency towards clotting). These are the familiar constituents of Metabolic Syndrome! They were present when the patient became insulin resistant, long before diabetes was diagnosed—in fact, 87% of diabetics are shown to have Metabolic Syndrome.

A recent study done in the US showed that people with diabetes and Metabolic Syndrome have the highest incidence of coronary artery disease, while people with diabetes without Metabolic Syndrome had the same prevalence of CAD as nondiabetics without Metabolic Syndrome.

Treatment of Diabetes

By now, it is clear that treatment of diabetes involves much more than control of blood sugar. However, the importance of controlling blood sugar must not be minimized.

To determine how well your diabetes is controlled, we monitor blood sugars and Hemoglobin A_{1C} (abbreviated $HgbA_{1C}$), a blood test usually performed in a laboratory. While testing for blood glucose is a way to tell what your sugars are on day-to-day basis, $HgbA_{1C}$ levels show how well the diabetes was controlled within the last 2–3 months. Both tests are useful and supplement each other. Ideally, blood glucose for diabetics should be under 120 mg/dl before meals and under 160 mg/dl after meals and before bedtime. The recommended glucose control by the American Diabetes Association is to have the level of $HgbA_{1C}$ below 7 percent; other organizations consider less than 6.5 percent more appropriate.

Diabetic patients check their blood sugar with a home glucose monitor and keep a logbook. Diabetics should check the glucose every morning (even if they are not taking insulin) and also frequently after meals (checking two hours after the meal is optimal).

The treatment of diabetes starts from learning about diabetes: what it is, how to eat, how to take care of yourself, what to expect from diabetes and how to live with it in an amicable way. Where would you start? Consultation with a certified diabetic educator (CDE) is a good way. This should be an advanced course when compared to the one you need to take about Metabolic Syndrome.

Diet and exercise should top the list of treatment options for diabetes. Those are actually not an option, they are necessity. As strange as it sounds, it is common that once the person finds out he has diabetes, he feels much better than before. The reason is that once diagnosed, a patient learns about diabetes and begins making lifestyle changes. The patients feel more energetic as blood sugar, which was up for a long time, goes down. Exercising regularly helps tremendously for psychological, as well as physical, wellbeing. We will talk about exercise and other lifestyle changes in the discussion of Metabolic Syndrome treatment.

When diet and exercise prove insufficient in achieving treatment goals, the usual next step is to proceed to glucose-lowering medications. As recently as 5 years ago, we had only 2 groups of medications to treat diabetes. Today, there are 6 groups of medications, each of which has its own place in the treatment of diabetes. This continuous progress is why medical books become quickly outdated—there is so much research in this area that the updates on books like this are needed every couple of years.

Some diabetes medications stimulate insulin release by the pancreas, including longer-acting drugs like glipizide, glyburide and glimepiride, as well as shorter acting drugs, such as repaglinide and nateglinide.

Metformin improves insulin resistance by decreasing glucose production in the liver. Rosiglitazone and pioglitazone improve insulin resistance by improving glucose uptake by the muscle and fat cells. These are newer insulin sensitizers, having replaced troglitazone, which was taken off the market because of rare cases of liver toxicity. Alpha glucosidase inhibitors (acarbose, miglitol) retard glucose uptake in the intestine. Finally, insulin (in its many forms) may be needed, usually in high doses for insulin-resistant Type 2 diabetics.

Why do we need so many medications? First, because diabetes is a complex disease involving insulin secretion (deficiency) and its action (resistance). Also, the natural history of diabetes is that, with time, the pancreas gets more and more exhausted, even with the help of medications. What was controlling the blood sugar last year does not work anymore this year. All these medications have different mechanisms of action, potency, safety profile and cost. Our discussion of diabetic medications has been greatly simplified; much more can be found on the American Diabetes Association website (www.diabetes.org) and in periodicals. The treatment of diabetes in each patient is individual, and each of the medications could be used singly or in combination, depending on the individual case.

All these treatments are good as long as they serve the goal, keeping the $HgbA_{1C}$ under control, recommended to be under 7 percent (or under 6.5 percent, depending on whom you ask). In real life, because of the continuous progression of diabetes, it is not unusual to take 2, 3, or even 4 different medications at the same time.

Treatment of diabetes is much more than treatment of high blood sugar. Medical care for a patient with diabetes involves treatment of many factors, including high blood sugar, high blood pressure, and unfavorable cholesterol. The feet should be inspected daily and checked every time you see the doctor. A yearly dilated eye exam is mandatory. Twice a year, a urinalysis is recommended. Once a year, the urine should also be checked for small amounts of albumin, a protein that may leak through the kidneys from the bloodstream.

All diabetics should be on aspirin unless there are specific reasons against its use, since it prevents clots from forming in diseased arteries. Blood pressure should not go above 135/85, and 120/70 would be far preferable. The tight control of blood pressure is also important for prevention of diabetic kidney disease.

Lipid profile should be optimized, keeping the LDL below 100mg/dl, HDL above 45 mg/dl (for men), or 55 mg/dl (for women), triglycerides under 150 mg/dl. (The LDL recommendations are identical to the recommendations for patients who have already had a heart attack).

Long-term studies with diabetics have shown that when one or more of these factors (blood sugar, blood pressure, increased clotting, or high cholesterol) is treated, then the rate of complications takes a dive. Many studies done in the US, Europe and Japan demonstrated a dramatic drop of the complication rate when people with diabetes are treated for any of the following: high blood pressure, high blood glucose or high cholesterol, when compared to diabetics who are not treated for these same risk factors.

These are new and important concepts: researchers in the United Kingdom Prospective Diabetes Study learned that death from cardiovascular cause in diabetics was dramatically decreased by controlling blood pressure, perhaps more significantly than by controlling blood sugar! Risk of stroke was decreased 44%, heart failure by 56% and diabetes-related death by 32%. Several large studies demonstrated significant lowering of cardiovascular risk (roughly 25% drop in risk) when high cholesterol in diabetics was aggressively controlled.

If you are already diagnosed with diabetes, you need a change of lifestyle, medications, and periodic examinations to prevent the development of complications of diabetes and coronary artery disease. But, please, look around you—your adult children and younger siblings are likely to be at an earlier stage of Metabolic Syndrome when diabetes is still *preventable.*

It takes a lot of effort from both the patient and the doctor. The payoff, however, is clear: fewer strokes, fewer heart attacks, fewer hospitalizations, fewer amputations, less eye damage, and a longer and better life.

3

Abnormal Cholesterol Profile—Dyslipidemia

Cholesterol is very commonly measured as part of a routine check-up because of its strong association with heart disease risk. For years, only total cholesterol was measured, and anything above 240 was considered high. As we learned more about atherosclerosis, now we check not only the cholesterol, but also its fractionation into different constituents called lipoproteins (HDL, LDL, or triglycerides, depending on their density). Using these markers, your physician can tell you if your pattern is likely to lead to heart disease.

The High Density Lipoprotein Cholesterol—HDL-C

The High Density Lipoprotein Cholesterol, or HDL-C, is the "good" cholesterol that helps keep the arteries from clogging. HDL-C below 35 mg/dl is considered to be a separate risk factor for CAD. Women, in general, have higher HDL levels than men do, so this number for women should be above 55 mg/dl, while men should have HDL-C above 45 mg/dl.

Low-Density Lipoprotein Cholesterol—LDL-C

Low-Density Lipoprotein Cholesterol, or LDL-C, is the "bad" cholesterol. This is the major cholesterol that clogs the arteries; the risk of a heart attack is increased with the increase of the LDL-C. Damage to the arteries is not necessarily permanent; if you bring your LDL-C down, the atherosclerotic plaques on the arteries may improve. The recommended LDL-C for people without any risk factors is below 160 mg/dl. For patients without known CAD, but with 2 risk factors (like family history and hypertension), the recommended LDL-C is below 130 mg/dl; for people with diabetes or known CAD the recommended level is below 100 mg/dl.

LDL-C is not just one homogenous molecule—it consists of small-dense and large-fluffy LDL-C. The small-dense LDL-C is the worst. These are small particles that more easily penetrate into the vessel wall and stick to it, making fatty plaques ready to rupture and cause a problem. The measurement of these particles is not readily available, but can be done in special labs.

The level of LDL-C is not a criterion for Metabolic Syndrome. However, patients with Metabolic Syndrome have been shown to have higher levels of the more dangerous small-dense LDL-C as a percentage of the total LDL-C. This can actually improve as Metabolic Syndrome is treated.

Triglyceride—TG

Triglyceride (TG) is another type of lipids that may contribute to form atherosclerotic disease. This type of fat is in abundance right after a fatty or high carbohydrate meal; that is why lipids should be checked in a fasting state. The higher the triglyceride level, the more likely the LDL-C is to have predominantly small-dense size. Thus, the triglyceride level is doubly important. Optimally, triglycerides should be below 150 mg/dl.

Total Cholesterol to HDL-C Ratio

A very important parameter is the total cholesterol to HDL-C ratio. People with this ratio under 3.5 have very low risk of CAD, while someone with the ratio above 6 is at a high risk. Consider someone with total cholesterol of 220 mg/dl. If the HDL is 30 mg/dl, that makes the ratio 7.3, suggesting high risk. And conversely, if the HDL is 85 mg/dl, the ratio is 2.6, which puts him at low risk for CAD.

Lipid Pattern in Metabolic Syndrome

The characteristic patterns of lipid abnormalities in people with Metabolic Syndrome involve elevated TG and low levels of HDL-C; total cholesterol and LDL-C may be low, normal or elevated. Because of the high triglyceride level, the LDL-C, regardless of its level, usually has a predominance of small-dense LDL-C.

Because of the low HDL-C, the total-C to HDL ratio is frequently high (above 6). All these make the pattern of lipids in Metabolic Syndrome highly atherogenic (promoting clogging of arteries). The association of insulin resistance and dyslipidemia is shown in multiple studies. The role of insulin resistance as the primary defect is also well demonstrated. Increased flux of free fatty acids into the liver, where cholesterol is made, is the major contributor to the specific lipid abnormalities (high TG, low HDL, and small-dense LDL-C) of Metabolic Syndrome. These lipid abnormalities (high TG, low HDL-C) are easily measured, and are the earliest manifestations of Metabolic Syndrome.

Lowering of LDL-C and TG, and raising of HDL-C is typically done with medications. Reduction of saturated fat and trans-fat in the diet plays a role in reducing LDL-C, while reduction of carbohydrate in the diet helps lower TG. Regular exercise and modest alcohol consumption may help raise HDL-C. Consumption of essential fatty acids (found in fish oil, flax seed oil, and hemp seed oil) may be of benefit.

In summary, the Metabolic Syndrome is associated with a specific pattern of lipid abnormalities including high triglycerides, low HDL-C and small-dense LDL-C, predisposing the individual for CAD. The dyslipidemia of insulin resistance is quite specific, it is rarely found in non-insulin-resistant individuals and it could be a first clue to the patient's being insulin resistant.

4

High Blood Pressure— Hypertension

Hypertension or high blood pressure is a common disease that becomes more prevalent with age. High blood pressure is a very well known risk factor for cardiovascular disease. A common myth we often hear is, "I feel well when my blood pressure is 160/100, so that is a good blood pressure for me." 160/100 is an elevated BP and is causing damage even if the person is feeling great. Multiple epidemiological studies throughout the world identified hypertension as a major risk factor for strokes and heart attacks. It is clear that blood pressure should be controlled to below 135/85 by any means necessary. What is less known is the association of blood pressure with insulin resistance and Metabolic Syndrome, although we do know that people with higher levels of insulin have twice as much chance of developing hypertension as non-insulin resistant people.

Can all types of hypertension be linked to insulin resistance? Definitely not. In some patients, hypertension is caused by diseases of kidneys, large arteries, adrenals, etc. Insulin resistance underlies hypertension of "unknown cause," the so-called essential hypertension, which is more common. These people usually have the other constituents of Metabolic Syndrome, including apple type obesity, dyslipidemia, glucose intolerance or diabetes. About 50% of people with essential hypertension have Metabolic Syndrome. The correlation of Metabolic Syndrome and hypertension is less strong in ethnic minorities.

Hyperinsulinemia may cause hypertension by different physiological mechanisms, including the way our body handles salt, causing structural changes in the vessels. Weight loss was commonly used as a first step treatment for hypertension. It works. What we are learning now is that the blood pressure lowering is likely mediated by improvement of insulin sensitivity. Weight reduction, particularly when combined with reduction in salt intake, alleviates insulin resistance and coincidentally, lowers blood pressure.

The goal in treatment of hypertension is to maintain the blood pressure below 135/85. It is important to remember about the beneficial effects of exercise and weight loss on blood pressure. There are numerous medications to lower blood pressure, and sometimes a combination of 2 or 3 drugs is necessary to keep the blood pressure under control. There are advantages to certain drugs in certain situations. For example, a group of medications called ACE inhibitors (angiotensin converting enzyme inhibitors) and ARBs (angiotensin receptor blockers) have shown additional benefit beyond simple lowering of blood pressure in reducing cardiovascular mortality.

PART II

The Stages and Features of Metabolic Syndrome

Wide is the range of words, on one side and the other.

—Homer

METABOLIC SYNDROME is not a disease, it is a prediabetic condition that may or may not develop into diabetes. Screening for Metabolic Syndrome is important because of its relationship with heart disease, hypertension and diabetes—people who have it are more likely to suffer a heart attack. Metabolic Syndrome can be recognized at a very early stage or after the person has had a heart attack or stroke.

Metabolic Syndrome is found at slightly higher rates in certain ethnic populations, mainly nonwhite populations. Genetics are important in the rates of transformation from predisease to overt disease.

Metabolic Syndrome goes hand in hand with a major cause of infertility in women, Polycystic Ovary Syndrome. Insulin resistance is a central feature of this condition.

5

Stages of Metabolic Syndrome

In matters of observation, chance favors only the prepared mind.

—Louis Pasteur

There are 3 presumptive stages of Metabolic Syndrome, each of which may last years or even decades. These stages could also be seen as severity levels.

The majority of people in the *first stage* are in their twenties or thirties. They are mildly or moderately overweight, with a round tummy, and may report a 10–20 pound weight gain since age 20. Often, there is a first-degree relative (parent or sibling) or other relative with adult onset diabetes. Biochemical testing usually demonstrates a characteristic cholesterol profile: low or low normal HDL and mild elevation of triglyceride; blood pressure and blood sugar are usually normal. This stage may be viewed as a "pre-prediabetic" stage.

In the *second stage* of Metabolic Syndrome, there could be additional features: high blood pressure (frequently only in the doctors office), impaired fasting glucose (IFG—fasting glucose level between 100-126), glucose intolerance (elevated blood sugar levels after eating), and a pronounced dyslipidemia. At this point, some people will already have coronary artery disease. This is a truly prediabetic stage.

The *third stage* is frank diabetes, with more chances of getting all the components of the syndrome. At this stage, there is additionally insulin deficiency, because the pancreas is no longer able to provide the high levels of insulin needed to compensate for the impaired insulin action. At this point, the treatment strategy remains the same, but with time, the treatment relies more heavily on medications, as the patient has now developed clinical diabetes.

As soon as you are aware that you may possibly have Metabolic Syndrome, start the lifestyle changes to improve the insulin action. It is possible and crucial to avoid progression from the early stage of Metabolic Syndrome to the late stage, so try to return to the previous stage instead of progressing to the next one.

6

Identifying Metabolic Syndrome

A simple questionnaire will help you determine whether you have Metabolic Syndrome. The following questions address genetic as well as acquired/lifestyle causes of Metabolic Syndrome.

Self-Assessment Quiz

1. Do you have a first degree relative (parent or sibling) with diabetes?
   Yes – 30 points   No – 0 points

2. Have you gained 20 or more pounds since age 20?
   Yes – 30   No – 0

3. Is your excess weight mostly distributed around your waist?
   Yes – 30   No – 0

4. Is your total cholesterol more than 200 mg/dl?
   Yes – 15   No – 0

5. Is your HDL cholesterol less than 40 mg/dl (men) or
   50 mg/dl (women)?
   Yes – 30   No – 0   Don't know – 15

6. How often do you eat fast food (French fries, fried meats, pepperoni pizza)?

   More than twice a week – 30   1–2 times weekly – 15
                          Less than once a week – 0

7. Do you belong to one of the following ethnic groups: Hispanic, American Indian, Asian Indian or African American?

   Yes – 15   No – 0

8. Do you spend more than 8 hours a day sitting (in the car, at work, at the computer, watching TV)?

   Yes – 30   No –0

9. Do you walk or exercise at least 1 hour per day?

   Yes – subtract 30   No – 15

10. Do you have gout?

    Yes – 30   No – 0

11. Do you have high blood pressure (systolic >135 mmHg/diastolic >85 mmHg)?

    Yes – 15   No – 0

12. Total Score: _____ points

Evaluation

If you scored:

- More than 105 points, you almost certainly have Metabolic Syndrome.

- 60 to 105 points, it is still likely that you have Metabolic Syndrome.

- 30 to 60 points, it is unlikely that you have Metabolic Syndrome.

- –30 to +30 points, you are in a good shape.

If you are taking medications for diabetes, high cholesterol and high blood pressure, there is no doubt that you have Metabolic Syndrome. The reason for this book is to identify individuals with early stages of Metabolic Syndrome.

If you have a first or second degree relative with diabetes, and you have gained about 20 pounds since age 20 (mostly around your belly), and you continue eating a mostly contemporary American diet and you hardly ever exercise, then you are at really high risk for Metabolic Syndrome.

If you have a hard time losing weight, have elevated blood pressure when you see your doctor, and have elevated triglyceride, and low HDL, your chances of having Metabolic Syndrome are quite high.

7

Syndrome X, Syndrome W, And Syndrome U

Syndrome X was described by Dr Gerald Reaven in 1988 and is the basis for Metabolic Syndrome. Dr Reaven is the founder of the basic concept of insulin resistance as the underlying cause for a constellation of metabolic abnormalities described in this book, as explained in the Introduction. With further research in large populations, the concept of Metabolic Syndrome has been refined.

Dr Harriet Mogul developed the concept of Syndrome W, which is a constellation of abdominal Weight gain, Waist size increase, and White-coat hypertension in middle aged Women. This is likely to be an early stage of Metabolic Syndrome.

What really matters is Syndrome U—You. Not all the individuals with Metabolic Syndrome will have all the constituents of Syndrome X or W. Everybody is unique, and none of these syndromes starts at one particular moment. When there is only one sign of the syndrome, e.g. mild obesity, decreased HDL-C or a tendency to have elevated blood pressure in the office, it is not always obvious that there is a pre-disease state requiring close attention and treatment. Most of the susceptible people would have one or two of the components of Metabolic Syndrome, but with aging, these will develop into a full-blown disease if not addressed. Age is a strong promoter of insulin resistance. As you know, age is also irreversible, making other constituents like obesity, dyslipidemia, hypertension and clotting the only treatable targets.

8

Ethnicity and Genetics in Metabolic Syndrome

People come in many billions
That's equal to a lot of millions
They also come in many colors
White, black, brown and many others
People come in all shapes and sizes
But what we need to realize is
We're all different, but that's OK
'Cause we're the same in other ways

—Elize Manoukian, 8 years old

Ethnicity unites groups of people with the same race, language and culture. All the ethnic groups are unique. They have their own cuisine, language, history and customs. We also know that people of the same ethnicity frequently share similar groups of genes not carried by other ethnic groups. This explains why many diseases occur frequently in some ethnic groups and are almost unheard of in others. Some of the diseases occur exclusively in people with a particular ethnicity. More commonly, diseases tend to occur more in one ethnic group than another. Insulin resistance and diabetes are among the best examples of how different the same disease or predisease can be, depending on your skin color. Some ethnic groups have more obesity (Mexican-Americans, African-Americans), some more hypertension (African-Americans). The rates of the complications are different in different groups, and so is the response to different medications. In any case, all of the ethnic groups in this country have high prevalence of insulin resistance that results in diabetes, which is a major problem for all countries in the world.

The United States is a *mixture of mixtures* of ethnic groups from throughout the world. If you are looking for an exotic restaurant, the US is a fine place to be. But if you are a physician, you need to be familiar with who is likely to get what disease or condition, depending what part of the world the patients' ancestors are from. Westernization and urbanization make things even more complicated. For instance, Japanese emigrating to the US develop less stomach cancer, but more coronary artery disease.

These are, of course, rough estimates. Asians are a very diverse group including Chinese, Vietnamese, Japanese, East Indians, Pakistanis, and

TABLE 4

Major Ethnic Segments of United States Population

Total Population	*268 million*
Caucasian	193 million
African-American	33 million
Indo-Hispanic	10 million
Euro-Hispanic	6 million
Afro-Hispanic	5 million
Asian	9 million
American Indian	2 million
Other	10 million

Source: *Diabetes Care* (1998, Sep). 21(9):1414-31.

many other ethnic groups that have completely different genetic predisposition for specific diseases. African-Americans vary immensely depending on the time of emigration and part of the Africa they are from. Bear with us as we lump some groups in order to make this as simple as possible.

The epidemiological data from the World Health Organization predicts a diabetes epidemic. In the world as a whole, between 1995 and 2025 the adult population will increase by 64%, prevalence of diabetes will increase by 35%, and the number of people with diabetes will increase by 122%. Table 5 shows the estimated number of adults with diabetes in different countries. The increase in cases of diabetes is worldwide, but interestingly, the developing countries will have a more dramatic increase in the new cases of diabetes.

TABLE 5

Top 10 Countries for Estimated Number (Millions) of Adults with Diabetes: 1995 and 2025

Rank	Country	1995 Millions	Country	2025 Millions
1	India	19.4	India	57.2
2	China	16.0	China	37.6
3	US	13.9	US	21.9
4	Russia	8.9	Pakistan	14.5
5	Japan	6.3	Indonesia	12.4
6	Brazil	4.9	Russia	12.2
7	Indonesia	4.5	Mexico	11.7
8	Pakistan	4.3	Brazil	11.6
9	Mexico	3.8	Egypt	8.8
10	Ukraine	3.6	Japan	8.5
	All other countries	49.7	All other countries	103.6
Total		135.3		300.0

Source: *Diabetes Care* (1998, Sep). 21(9):1414-31.

As you can see, Asian Indians clearly are very susceptible to diabetes. They have a 2–3 times higher incidence of diabetes and 4 times higher incidence of CAD than non-Hispanic whites. Even though general obesity is not common in Asian Indians, the central distribution of the weight is very common. The migrant Asian Indians have increased mortality from CAD in the United Kingdom when compared with Europeans, likely related to their higher prevalence of diabetes.

In US, the prevalence of diabetes is highest in Pima Indians, 50% in their general population, and 70–80% of people older than 60. In general, non-white ethnic groups are more susceptible to insulin resistance, obesity and diabetes than whites. In the 65–74 year old age group, the prevalence of diabetes was 33% in Hispanics (Mexican-Americans, Cuban-Americans, and Puerto Ricans) compared with 17% in non-Hispanic whites.

Mexican Americans and Asian Indians have higher predisposition to the Metabolic Syndrome. Overall, 25% of whites, 22% of African Americans, and 32% of Mexican Americans were classified as having Metabolic Syndrome.

The genetics of Metabolic Syndrome are poorly understood. Genes possibly linked to Metabolic Syndrome have been identified on several chromosomes. A common set of genes may determine not only fasting insulin levels, but also lipid and obesity traits. Studies involving identical twins show that if one twin has Metabolic Syndrome, the other twin has a 50% chance of having Metabolic Syndrome.

Genes are very important in determining Metabolic Syndrome. However, over the past half century, increased sedentary lifestyle and unlimited access to Calories have blossomed the genes of insulin resistance into an epidemic of Metabolic Syndrome.

9

Polycystic Ovary Syndrome (PCOS)

Polycystic ovary syndrome (PCOS) is a leading cause of infertility in women in the US. Approximately 5 million women in the US suffer from this disorder, 6-10% of women of reproductive age. Young women with PCOS commonly seek medical attention because of irregular menstrual periods, obesity, infertility, excessive hair growth (hirsutism), adolescent acne and male-pattern hair thinning. More than 65% of women with PCOS are overweight, with a body mass index above 27. The fat distribution is usually of abdominal pattern. Most often symptoms appear in adolescence around the start of menstruation. However, some women do not develop symptoms until their mid-20s. Variations in manifestation of the disease are largely dependent on the ethnicity of the person. Obesity is more common in Hispanic women; hair growth is less pronounced in Asian women.

The symptoms in PCOS are caused by elevation of male hormones (such as testosterone) in women. Multiple small cysts appear on the ovaries, stimulated by high insulin levels in the blood. Infertility is caused by anovulation, when there is no egg release from the ovaries available for conception. Irregular menstrual periods frequently characterized by delayed and heavy flow are typical for anovulation. Some women will miss their menstrual periods for several months or years at a time.

Within the last decade, it has been shown that PCOS is an insulin resistant state and too much insulin is the likely cause of testosterone overproduction by the ovaries. High levels of testosterone interfere with pituitary function leading to anovulation, amenorrhea (missed periods) and infertility.

Frequently, women with PCOS have impaired glucose tolerance. PCOS is a manifestation of Metabolic Syndrome in young women—30% develop diabetes by age 30. The dyslipidemia of insulin resistance is commonly found in PCOS women, and these women are at increased risk of developing CAD, just like people with Metabolic Syndrome.

When insulin resistance improves, either due to weight loss or medication, women can get pregnant. It has been shown that even a 10–15% weight reduction resulted in spontaneous conception in about 75% of obese women with PCOS. There is growing evidence of beneficial use of insulin-sensitizing agents, like metformin and glitazones (pioglitazone and rosiglitazone) on PCOS.

PART III

Treatment of Metabolic Syndrome

*Keeping your body healthy is an expression of gratitude to
the whole cosmos—the trees, the clouds, everything.*

—Thich Nhat Hanh

MUCH OF the attention to diabetes over the past decades has
focused on the development of new treatments. We now have
a variety of new medications and better diagnostic tools to help patients;
however, treatment of diabetes remains difficult and costly. It is much
more logical and cost effective to prevent the diabetes by treating people
with Metabolic Syndrome, viewed as a precursor to diabetes. More than
80% of people with diabetes have Metabolic Syndrome—diabetes that
could have been prevented in these people. The earlier this prevention
starts, the more chance the person has of avoiding not only diabetes, but
also heart disease. 50% of people with CAD have Metabolic Syndrome.
Long before they developed the CAD, they had Metabolic Syndrome.

Is there any evidence that treating Metabolic Syndrome will *prevent* diabetes or CAD? Within the last 2–3 years, multiple studies from around the world have shown that making changes in lifestyle could prevent diabetes from developing in people with impaired fasting glucose.

The Diabetes Prevention Program (DPP), a study done in the US, included 3,234 people at risk for developing diabetes. They were enrolled in 3 groups: lifestyle modification, medication (using metformin), and a control group that did not receive any specific instructions. The lifestyle change protocol included weekly sessions on diet, increased physical activity up to 150 minutes per week, and the goal that participants lose 7% of their initial weight. At the end of the study, there was a significant 58% reduction in developing diabetes in the lifestyle group. Metformin is a medication that helps improve insulin resistance by reducing glucose outflow from the liver. In the group taking metformin, the risk reduction was less robust, 31% compared to controls. Both interventions worked, but when compared, lifestyle changes were more effective than medicine in decreasing the risk of development of diabetes. A similar study was done in Finland and was called the Diabetes Prevention Study. Lifestyle changes in this study included body weight reduction of at least 5%, reduced dietary fat intake (<30% of total Calories), reduced saturated fat intake (<10% of total Calories), increased dietary fiber (>15 g/100 Cal) and increased aerobic exercise (to 30 minutes per day). The result for the Finnish study was exactly the same as in the DPP study: 58% risk reduction of diabetes in all of the groups and even a whopping 65% reduction in those who followed all four lifestyle changes.

In another study (San Antonio, Texas), it was shown that preventing normal individuals from becoming overweight would result in the greatest reduction in incidence of Type 2 diabetes. This would result in a 62 and 74% reduction in the incidence of Type 2 diabetes in Mexican Americans and non-Hispanic whites, respectively. Preventing the entire population from gaining, on average, 1 unit of body mass index (BMI) would result in a reduction in incidence of Type 2 diabetes of 12.4 and 13.0% in Mexican Americans and non-Hispanic whites, respectively.

Preliminary data from Sweden suggest that the use of orlistat (fat absorption blocker) in combination with lifestyle changes prevented diabetes by 37%, compared with lifestyle changes alone when used in patients with impaired fasting glucose. A similar trial in Canada using acarbose (carbohydrate absorption blocker) showed a 25% risk reduction in development of diabetes, which was in turn was associated with a 49% risk reduction in development of cardiovascular disease.

Now we know that the onset of diabetes is preventable. More studies are in progress to see if heart disease is preventable in the same population. We will get the definitive answers in several years. Meanwhile, let's work on lifestyle changes.

10

Diet That is Acceptable

Thou shouldst eat to live, not live to eat.
—Socrates

The Webster Dictionary defines diet as a prescribed course of what is to be eaten and what is not. We are going to expand this definition. We will include food choices that are good and bad, and in addition to these "dos and don'ts" of food, we'll discuss a change in thinking about food and a way of eating.

We will try to limit the use of the terms "good" and "bad." The punitive implications of a food being "bad" are an unnecessary distraction. Think in terms of whether the food is going to give you the desired result. Will potato chips give you your desired result? What is *your* desired result?

Perhaps the main goal of the diet is to live a healthy life. A gradual change in your lifestyle will improve the profile of your risk factors and lower your risk for diabetes, Metabolic Syndrome and CAD. Even if you do not have any risk factors for these metabolic diseases, the healthy diet is still important. If you make changes in your diet, it will also decrease your risk for certain cancers. Certain fats, food coloring and preservatives are suspected causes of migraine headaches, breast and colon cancer,

Alzheimer's disease and many others. This chapter is about a healthy way of eating, and all members of your family, particularly children, will greatly benefit from it.

Weight loss is a common goal of dieting because of the way you may look and feel. Even with modest weight loss, you will see major benefits, such as blood pressure improvement and better diabetic control. Even if you do not need to lose weight, there may be room to improve your eating habits for multiple other reasons. If, in the case of an exercise program "anything" works, the weight loss program should not be "anything that will make you lose weight." Crash diets have been shown to be worthless—it just takes a short while to regain the weight, frequently even more than was lost. The body requires a variety of food constituents, micronutrients, minerals, vitamins and activity to run smoothly.

Bookstores are filled with books about diets, such as the Atkins diet, Zone Diet, Protein Power, low fat diets (American Heart Association, Ornish's diet) and the low glycemic diet. Dieting is not easy, particularly considering the diversity of ethnic cultures. The epidemic of obesity and its consequences has dictated the need for creating new approaches to the way we eat. The above-mentioned diets all brought some new ideas into meal planning. Low carbohydrate, high protein, low fat diets are successful in achieving certain goals, although some features of these diets can be harmful when followed to extreme. It is also not easy to stay on these diets, and weight frequently bounces back when the person goes back to his or her usual eating habits.

Dr Reaven recommends the Syndrome X diet for treatment of insulin resistance and prevention of diabetes. The main emphasis of this diet is the proportion of protein:fat:carbohydrate ratio of 15%:40%:45%. This is based on his research that diets low in carbohydrate and high in monounsaturated fats are improving the insulin levels and the dyslipidemia (high triglycerides and low HDL) of insulin resistance. Of the 40% of Calories coming from fat, $1/4$ or less should come from saturated fat. (In other words, 10% or less of the total Calories should come from saturated fat.)

Now let's define Calories. A calorie is the amount of energy needed to heat 1 cc of water by 1 degree Centigrade. A food calorie, which is capitalized to Calorie, equals 1000 calories, or 1 kilocalorie (1 kcal). It is the amount of energy needed to heat 1000 cc of water by one degree Centigrade. Energy content of food is expressed as Calories. Thus a small potato might contain 100 Calories, or 100 kcal. When burned, this energy will raise the temperature of 100 *kilo*grams of water (i.e., a 220 lb human) by 1 degree Centigrade. If not burned, it will be stored as roughly 9 grams (two teaspoons) of fat.

What is the problem with the American diet? We eat too much, and too much of that is unhealthy food. The main characteristics of "the American diet" are large quantity and poor quality. Sugared beverages and high fat snacks are available without much effort or financial stretch.

"Turn Back the Calendar" Diet

The diet that is recommended in this book is a universal healthy diet with emphasis on types of fat, types of carbohydrates, amount of fiber, artificial additives, food coloring, etc. The portions are crucial and will decrease spontaneously, because healthy meals are satisfying and do not cause food cravings.

If we have to name our diet it will be "Turn Back the Calendar," because it reflects the way people used to eat half a century ago. We are not trying to preach so much living in the past as selectively undoing the present. The best part is that, with suggested food choices, you get to ignore most everything that is advertised on TV.

The Great Eating Scam

How do you suppose humans have eaten through the ages? Do you suppose they ate meat every day? Do you suppose your ancestors ate fried potatoes? Candy? Gatorade? Diet Coke? How often do you think they ate pizza, chocolate, ice cream, or white bread? For how many generations has your family owned a refrigerator? Did they drink milk or orange juice every day? Did they eat bananas "because they're supposed to have lots of potassium"?

In our clinic, we have a substantial geriatric population. We asked the sharpest eighty- and ninety-year olds (interestingly most of them are women): "What did you eat throughout your life?" The answer was almost always the same, ". . . lots of vegetables and fruits and some meat . . . " (none were vegetarian, by the way). They don't eat fast foods and they minimize snacks. Many were given cod liver oil as children. They look thin, healthy, energetic and bright.

The twentieth century is not only famous because people walked on the moon, but also for new, incredible techniques of food production and new ways of influencing people to buy, eat, and buy again. In the US more than anywhere else, commercialization created fast food chains, high Calorie snacks, frosted cereals, hydrogenation of fats to make the food live forever and high carbohydrate drinks. Things that do not belong in the diet appeared, like hydrogenated fats, food colorings and daily desserts.

Here's a humorous, but blatant, example. Dry cat food is often artificially colored. Cats happen to be colorblind. They most likely don't care if their dinner is brightly colored; the coloring is strategically added to influence the pet's owner. Does it belong there? It's debatable. Most likely there is no harm done. Even if the additives posed a small risk, cats are still, excuse me, cheap and plentiful.

Let's take it to the next level. Do we need bright colors (however safe) on our M&Ms (which all taste the same, regardless of color) or on our kid's birthday cake (which is too sweet to eat anyway)? Do we need Yellow No. 5 (which asthmatics will fondly recognize as the asthma trigger, tartrazine) in our soft drinks? (Sushi lovers score extra credit for finding Yellow No. 5-free wasabi powder.) Does food coloring really belong in our toothpaste, our deodorant, our dishwashing soap, laundry detergent . . . ?

Welcome to the Great Eating Scam. Successful marketing depends on delivery of a uniform product. The folks out there know that you'll pay inflated prices for cheap products if they offer you something you've tasted/smelled/seen before. You'll head to McDonald's (marshmallow buns and Secret Sauce) before you take a risk with "Stan's Burger Joint" around the corner, off the beaten path. If unnecessary food additives become "necessary" to conceal minor variations in the natural color or flavor of the product, then so be it. Salty and sweet flavors, and crunchy texture let you know you're in familiar territory, you're still part of the club. Oil and grease act as effective solvents to deliver the flavor you want, when you want it (immediately).

And suddenly, it makes sense. Orange drink replaces orange juice. Crystal lemon drink replaces lemonade. Bacon has "smoky flavor" as a listed ingredient, and your toothpaste gel is beautiful blue. Predictable. Familiar.

To Eat or Not To Eat

Do we live to eat or eat to live? This question is a crucial one. Think about it frequently. People who live to eat may be drawn to high-fat meals that deliver instant flavor. They might like salty or sugary foods that satisfy inner cravings. They might like a variety of recipes.

People who eat to live might choose easily digestible foods; they might strive for moderation. They might select a vegetable for its taste, as opposed to how it tastes when smothered in cheese or dressing. They would certainly look for variety in their meals.

In fact, most of us do both. Nobody said that a healthy meal has to be bland or uninteresting. Nobody said that "living to eat" must include fast food. Remember that taste is an acquired feature. It comes with habit and culture and changes with practice and ability to overcome mental barriers. If up until now you ate only what you like, then, for the most part, you live to eat.

3 Easy Steps on the Way to New Thinking

STEP 1 Just Say "No" to Food You Know Is Basically
Unhealthy.

There is no sincerer love than love of food.

—George Bernard Shaw

Even if you love them to death, say "No" to the foods you know are
unhealthy. The "No, thanks" should not be for just now, a month, or a
diet course. The "No" should be for today, 3 months later, and 5 years
from now. Eat the same way at home, at work, during travel.

As confusing as it is, the less you eat, the less you want to eat. This
is very true about carbohydrates. When we eat carbohydrates, e.g., cookies, candies, or sweet juices, it causes production of more insulin, which
make us even hungrier. Breaking this cycle by saying "No" to the sweets
will make a big difference. We all recognize the times when we eat that
first potato chip, that first piece of chocolate, that first piece of bread from
the basket at the restaurant. Many times we don't remember the rest of
the bag of potato chips, the next five pieces of chocolate, the rest of the
basket. This "automatic eating" is often governed by insulin and is ampli-
fied in insulin-resistant persons.

To be fair, there is much more at play in determining what and how
much we eat. For example, dietary protein has an appetite-suppressing
effect, as does ketosis, a condition produced when fats and protein are
used for energy during fasting or starvation. Acknowledging these other
factors, the notion of carbohydrates causing hunger is still an exceedingly
useful concept. The successful "graduation" from the first step of learning to manage carbohydrate intake includes elimination of candy, jelly-
beans, juices, sodas (regular and diet alike), colorful sweet drinks in your
house and from the restaurant menu. Take them off your shopping lists
forever. Dispense with the other "dispensable carbohydrates," such as

potatoes, white bread, white rice, cornstarch and pasta made from refined grain.

STEP 2   Create New Meal Plans Using Your Imagination and New Ingredients.

> *The discovery of a new dish does more for human happiness than the discovery of a new star.*
>
> —Anthelm Brillat-Savarin

There are many, many ingredients out there waiting for you to discover and include in your gastronomic repertoire. Whole grains. Oats. Brown rice. Dried beans and lentils. Garbanzo beans. Nuts and seeds. Soy hot dogs. Tofu. Seitan. Shiitake mushrooms. Collard greens. Swiss chard. Spinach. Beets. These can be used as main courses, condiments, for variety, for flavor. With time, you get more used to healthy meals (brown rice instead of white rice, buckwheat noodles instead of semolina noodles, tofu instead of meat). Actually, eating meat is not bad at all—except that the meat should be chosen from animals that are raised in friendly conditions, such as chickens raised free of cages and cattle allowed to graze on open pastures. (Animals raised under these less crowded conditions carry fewer harmful bacteria and have a more favorable fatty acid content. They are also likely to contain less antibiotics.)

After creating a new way of eating, the thought about your previous way of eating will seem strange. "Ah, how could I have liked to eat that?" If you are doing the grocery shopping, then you need to change your shopping list, read labels, and maybe even change stores if you cannot find the right produce.

STEP 3   Set Limits for the Types of Food You Eat.

Good habits result from resisting temptation.

—Ancient Proverb

This is a very important step and should be done ASAP. You want to learn to control food cravings, the desire to eat, eat, and eat. Frequently, we will finish a whole bag of potato chips, go after the third serving of ribs, eat the third piece of See's candy, a bag of M&Ms, or a second piece of cake. A 16-ounce steak can be eaten by a family, instead of by one person. Most of the time, there is a mental fight between your subconscious wish for flavor (and desire not to waste food) and your conscious understanding that "this is not healthy."

As you reach for the second helping, let the voice-tape play in your head, "Humans are the only species that eat when they are not hungry."

Recognizing this conflict will help you overcome the cravings and self-destructive eating patterns. Once you realize that your health depends on what and how much you eat, you can do it. Setting limits on what you eat and how much is the main goal of this step. After a short time, you realize that cravings disappear and there is no problem stopping after a small piece of cake, or even turning down an offered See's candy. Adding some protein to your meals may be helpful, and this will be discussed in detail.

This mentality has worked for many people who quit smoking. The reason most of the people have given for stopping smoking is concern about their health. 40-50 years ago, people did not know about the hazards of smoking and many have died from lung cancer and emphysema. Once smoking became known as the main cause of lung cancer, many smokers quit.

There is ample evidence in the medical literature about the role of unhealthy diets on the development of diabetes, obesity and heart disease. It is time for the public to learn about that and quit unhealthy eating habits.

A Basic Lesson in Energy Balance

There are multiple formulas for calculation of the daily Calorie requirements. This is one of them:

Total Calories = Metabolic needs + physical exercise + fat storage

Briefly, what you eat is used for one of three purposes. You're either going to use it to make something (grow skin, hair; make enzymes, hormones, protein), burn it as fuel, or store it as fat. For the record, it's not quite that simple, but let's pretend it is.

The importance of this equation is that if you are obese, then two things can change it. Either you have to decrease the Calorie intake, or you should increase the physical activity to burn the Calories. We'll assume your metabolic needs are constant; again it's not quite that simple.

If you are overweight, then most likely you are overeating carbohydrates and fats. Most of the Calories come from fats and carbohydrates. Both carbohydrates and fats are stored as fat, if not needed for one of the other two functions. So, the goal of balanced eating is to maintain weight (if the weight is normal) or decrease weight (if you are overweight). This is done through a diverse meal plan with enough protein, fiber, fat and nutrients, avoiding high fat, high-refined carbohydrate meals. This should be done today, tomorrow, and in the future for you and all your family.

General Principles of a Healthy Diet

There is no healthy diet that would fit and satisfy everybody, but we should define some general principles. What are the things in the diet that make people gain weight and increase tendency for Metabolic Syndrome, diabetes, hypertension and CAD? *Those are certain fatty foods and certain carbohydrates.*

There are 3 main nutrients and 3 sources of energy: protein, fat and carbohydrates. We use protein for its structural value. It is less important as an energy source. We use fat and carbohydrates for structural and other purposes, and they are also recognized as prime sources of energy. So, we definitely need proteins, carbohydrates and fats that are transformed into Calories; the question is what kinds and how much.

Protein

Protein contains 4 Calories per gram. Its value, however, comes not from its use as fuel, but from its use as a structural building-block for our bodies. Those building-blocks include the unique chemical structures called amino acids. There are many kinds of amino acids. Our bodies use twenty of them to build proteins, for growing tissue, making enzymes, and other important uses. Eight of these amino acids are called "essential amino acids," because our bodies cannot manufacture them; we need to get them from food (or else we'll die). (There is a ninth essential amino acid, histidine, required for infants but not adults.)

We refer to any protein containing all eight of these essential amino acids as a "complete" protein. Animal products (meat, fish, poultry, eggs, milk, escargot, shellfish . . .) contain all of these eight essential amino acids.

Plant-based proteins typically are missing one or more of these eight essential amino acids. It is like a Scrabble set that is missing one or more letters. The trick to using plant-based proteins, as we will see, is to combine different plant groups (such as beans and grains).

Many plant-based products have the same protein content as animal products. Protein from animal sources is mixed with water, fat and cholesterol. Protein from vegetable sources comes mixed with fiber, and varying amounts of carbohydrates (beans, lentils, mushroom) or fat (nuts, seeds).

Cholesterol is only found in animal-based products; plants do not contain cholesterol. Vitamin B_{12} is also found in animal products; plant sources of this very important vitamin are rare.

Adequate protein intake is important. It is needed to build your body (hair, nails, bone matrix, cell membranes, enzymes, etc.). From a weight-control perspective, protein is shown to give us a feeling of satiety. Adequate protein intake also means you are eating less fat and carbohydrate.

The typical daily requirement for protein usually varies from 0.6–1.0 gram per kilogram of body weight, depending on age or health condition. Too much or too little protein could each cause health problems. Too little protein would halt growth and healing. Too much protein is hard on the digestive tract and kidneys. Excess protein can also cause calcium loss from bones, particularly in vulnerable older people. If the protein comes from meat and contains saturated fats, then an excess translates to hardening of the arteries.

Typically, it is recommended to obtain 12–20% of daily caloric intake from protein. The typical caloric intake for an adult should be about 1200–2000 Calories. 15% would be 180–300 Calories coming from protein, which comes to 45–75 grams of protein daily. This amount of protein is contained in roughly 6-10 ounces of meat. Many of our patients who get most of their protein from animal sources fall short of this daily intake of meat. What should they do? Increasing their meat intake will be hard to digest and might damage their kidneys or coronary arteries.

Here's the fun part. There are many plant foods with a protein content rivaling meat (20-25%). These include nuts, seeds, soy products and beans. Thus, a handful of (shelled) sunflower or pumpkin seeds can easily contain 5–10 grams of protein. A soy hot dog can easily contain 9 grams of protein. Tofu contains twice the protein ounce-for-ounce as egg white. We cheated a bit with the numbers; the protein content of beans is based on dry weight, while the protein content of meat is based on fresh meat and the water contained therein. Don't get caught up in the details.

Suddenly the diet becomes simple. I don't need to become a pure vegetarian for the sake of reducing saturated fat intake. 3–5 ounces of meat or fish with some additional protein coming from eggs, whole-grain bread, legumes and nuts would cover well for the structural needs of the body. A handful of sunflower seeds or nuts thrown over a bowl of oatmeal transforms a high-protein grain into a meal rivaling eggs or sausage as a segment of my daily protein needs.

In our practice, we have had some success by helping patients recognize protein sources from non-animal sources. Dried beans, lentils, tofu, soy hot dogs, almonds, sunflower seeds, pumpkin seeds, seitan and tempeh each contain about 20–25 percent protein. This is the same percentage as with animal sources, meat, fish, and chicken. Whole grains weigh in at 8–14 percent protein, comparable to eggs (12%). Mushrooms and seaweed are also very useful protein sources. Raw hulled pumpkin and sunflower seeds are available in bulk from many health food stores. They are easily dry-roasted in a pan on your stovetop.

Nuts and seeds are great additions to the daily meals. They can be added to the salads, cereal and breads. They contain fats, which happen to be unsaturated, and can improve your cholesterol, in contrast to the saturated fats found in meat.

A Word about Soy. Recently, there is a debate whether increased intake of soy products is associated with increased risk of mental decline, such as Alzheimer's disease. There are conflicting data, with other studies showing a significant protective effect of soy in preventing Alzheimer's disease. Soy may also have a place in treating menopausal symptoms.

There is wide concern about genetically modified crops, and soybeans are one of the crops that are most widely subjected to genetic modification. These modifications include the introduction of other plant, animal or bacterial genes into crops for specific effects. We recommend the use of organically produced soy and other crops. We would also push for laws mandating that genetically modified crops be labeled as such.

Fats

Contrary to some beliefs, fat is an important nutrient. We need fat to insulate our body, to make some hormones and to absorb certain vitamins (A, D, E and K) from the intestines. Fat is also a concentrated source of energy at 9 Calories per gram. What kind of fats are we talking about?

Fat and oil are basically the same thing (oil is liquid at room temperature and fat is solid at room temperature). There are monounsaturated, polyunsaturated and saturated fats that come from animals or plants. There are also trans fats and cholesterol.

Monounsaturated fats are the healthiest for the heart and cholesterol levels. Monounsaturated fatty acids or MUFA are the main constituent of olive oil. Canola oil and peanut oil and certain nuts also contain preferentially monounsaturated fats. It is well known that, traditionally, people consuming a Mediterranean diet have lower rates of heart disease—the Mediterranean diet is a high monounsaturated fat diet because everything is cooked or dressed with olive oil. The studies comparing high MUFA diets with the traditional American diet showed dramatic differences, including better patterns of insulin sensitivity, cholesterol profiles and weight. High MUFA diets lower bad LDL-cholesterol without harming levels of good HDL-cholesterol. In contrast, very low-fat diets have shown very modest and transient weight reduction, with a decrease in HDL or "good" cholesterol. The moral of the story: Don't try to eliminate fats completely, because they are important.

Polyunsaturated fats are found in vegetable oils, canola oil, flax oil, peanut butter, almond butter and fish oil. As it turns out, unsaturated fats tend to be associated with lower cholesterol, when compared with saturated fats.

Saturated fats tend to be solid at room temperature. The major sources of saturated fats are butter, lard, ghee, meats (beef, pork, chicken, lamb), dairy, coconut oil, and pastry made from butter or chocolate. Margarine also contains significant levels of saturated fats, but is to be condemned for other reasons (see the discussion on trans fats, below). *Cholesterol* frequently is present with these fats, but can also be found separately, such as in egg yolk.

Trans fats are unknown to nature. These are created in the lab under high temperatures, by reintroduction of hydrogen atoms into fatty acid chains, causing double bonds to randomly convert into single bonds. This process is called hydrogenation and many foods on the market contain *hydrogenated or partially hydrogenated fats.* These fats contain trans fatty acids. Trans fats are the worst fats healthwise. You can't (or at least shouldn't) use them the way we usually use fats (to build cell membranes, nerve coating, hormones). They are the main culprits of weight gain; they raise the bad LDL-C and lower the good HDL-C.

These partially hydrogenated fats give foods the properties of long shelf life. If you buy pastries made with these compounds and accidentally lose them in the back of your cupboard, you will note that they still appear fresh months and years later. Processed foods—margarine, snack foods, French-fries, shortenings and cheap baked goods, are main sources of trans fats. Previously thought to be harmless (remember when margarine was "better" than butter?), these trans fats are shown to harden the arteries and express other harmful effects (like suppression of immunity) on the body. The direct correlation has been shown between the eaten hydrogenated fat and body fat.

Having said that, *What should we eat? **Meat, poultry, fish, oils.***

A lot of patients say, " We eat much less meat than we used to." Still, the consumption of meat in this country is growing. "I don't eat meat— I eat lots of fish and chicken," people claim proudly. Is it okay to eat meat at all? Of course it is, but we should do some thinking around it.

First, choose lean cuts of meats. Lean red meat and chicken have a similar amount of fat. $^1/_2$ of a chicken breast without skin is 142 Calories, 3 oz of broiled lean lamb loin chop is 160 Calories, 3 oz of veal lean shoulder is 145 Calories, and 3 oz of lean round eye roasted is 156 Calories. There is really not a big difference, as you can see.

Second, it is crucial to watch your portions. Hardly ever does anyone admit eating $^1/_2$ of a chicken breast; it is not really that hard to cut it into two pieces. It is more important to stick with lean meats and small portions than to focus on what kind of meat you are going to eat.

Third, stay away from animals raised in crowded conditions. The fat percentage is much higher in these animals than in free raised animals. Natural so-called "free range chicken" is widely available in health food stores. The modestly increased price is probably well worth it. If you cut your portions in half, you will still save money. Raising chickens under crowded conditions makes them fat and depressed. If you eat these chickens, you will become fat and depressed. What do you expect?

Fourth, eat fish. The oils from certain fish are felt to be beneficial and have actually been used in treating many different diseases. The original evidence comes from Eskimos, whose main food is fish; the percentage of fat in their diet is about 70% and CAD is unheard of. What is protecting their hearts? There is solid evidence that certain oils that are found in the fish have anti-atherogenic (lowering cholesterol), anti-thrombotic (anti-clotting), and anti-inflammatory effects. These are omega-3 fatty acids that are (along with omega-6 fatty acids) also called essential fatty acids or EFAs. Essential means that our body needs them for health, and because you cannot make them, we need them in our diet.

Docosahexaenoic acid (DHA) and Eicosapentaenoic acid (EPA) are two omega-3 fatty acids found in the fish and fish oil. DHA is responsible for the trimming of cardiovascular risk. DHA is also shown to improve the blood pressure and heart rate.

Do all fish contain same amount of omega-3 fatty acids? The amount of omega-3 fatty acid per serving varies with the fish species and geography. Fish themselves obtain the omega-3 fatty acids from plankton (the EFAs are essential for the fish, too!). In general, the colder the water, the higher the omega-3 content of the fish that live in it. One hundred grams (a little over 3 ounces) of free-swimming Atlantic salmon contains 3-4 grams of omega-3 fatty acids, 40–50% of which is DHA. Farmed fish does not contain the same amount of beneficial fish oil, because it does not have access to the cold water plankton enjoyed by their wild counterparts.

Tuna, sardines, mackerel and herring are also DHA rich species. 100 grams of salmon (about 3 ounces) daily for 2–4 weeks showed a cardiovascular benefit. It is hard to eat fish every day, but 1–3 servings a week is not hard to do at all.

As you've probably heard, there can be problems with eating fish. Farm-raised fish may contain antibiotics or other toxins. Fish farming can be harmful to the coastal environment. Wild-caught fish may contain mercury, particularly fish high on the food chain such as swordfish and shark.

Is there any other important source of omega-3 fatty acid?

Flax oil or flaxseed oil is a very rich source of omega-3 fatty acid or linolenic acid. Flax oil contains omega-3 or linolenic acid, omega-6 or linoleic acid and omega-9 or oleic acid in proportions of 65%–18%–16%. When included in the diet, flax oil or crushed flaxseeds exhibit multiple beneficial effects, including improvement of cholesterol profile and anti-inflammatory processes, as well as improved work of the digestive system.

Flax is an annual plant grown mostly in the colder regions of the world. Flax oil breaks down at room temperature, which is why it is stored in the refrigerator section in supermarkets. Use it fresh out of the bottle onto your food! Cooking defeats the purpose of flax oil by breaking down the heat-sensitive essential fatty acids (and makes the flax oil taste like paint). Mixed with balsamic or plum vinegar, it can be a competitive salad dressing. Flaxseeds can be ground up and sprinkled on a salad or cereal, another good way of introducing yourself to flax oil. If you are pure vegetarian, then flax oil is even more important.

Another oil to consider is hemp seed oil, which contains large amounts of omega-6 and omega-3 fatty acids in a ratio that is useful to our bodies. Canola and vegetable oils also contain some omega-3 fatty acids, but in less favorable proportions of essential and other unsaturated fatty acids.

Rules for Protein and Fat Intake

In summary, we should read labels and know what we are eating. Just low fat is not good enough anymore. Follow these rules:

1. Avoid hydrogenated or partially hydrogenated fat by reading labels. Avoid margarine and "vegetable shortening" for the same reason.

2. Decrease intake of animal fat (high in cholesterol and saturated fat) by cutting down on portions and choosing lean cuts. Substitute meat with tofu or other high-protein plant sources when you can.

3. Eat fish (not farmed) 1–3 times per week.

4. Use olive oil as the main cooking oil. Use flaxseed oil fresh from the bottle.

5. Avoid fast food, which is extremely rich in hydrogenated and saturated fats.

6. If you are vegetarian, make sure you get enough protein and essential fatty acids.

7. If you are a meat eater, try to have some vegetarian days (1–3) per week, cut down on the portions (no more than 3 oz), choose lean cuts of red meat or chicken, and eat fish (rich in omega-3 fatty acids) 1–3 days a week.

Carbohydrates, Starches, Fiber

Just like fats, there are different types of carbohydrates. There are simple carbohydrates and complex carbohydrates or starches. The simple carbohydrates are mostly obtained from sugar, candy, juices, fruits, and sodas. These taste sweet, are easy to absorb, and momentarily increase the blood sugar.

The complex carbohydrates include starchy foods. Main sources of starches include breads, rice, pasta, any grains, potatoes and cereal. The body breaks down this starch into simple sugars as it is absorbed from the intestine.

The amount of insulin secreted by the pancreas depends on the amount and type of carbohydrate in the meal, and is affected by the rate at which the carbohydrate is absorbed. Low glycemic-index foods are digested more slowly and induce less insulin secretion. There is data that slowly absorbed, low glycemic-index foods (wheat bran, barley, oats, grainy breads made with whole seeds, lentils, kidney beans and garbanzo beans) are associated with increased HDL, help people lose weight, improve insulin sensitivity and reduce risk of diabetes.

As an analogy for glycemic index, imagine an accounting department at a factory. If the money trickles in slowly throughout the year, one accountant might be able to keep all the books. If all the money for the year comes in over a few days or weeks, then a larger team of accountants will be needed. Your pancreas needs to secrete a lot more insulin in response to a sudden load of sugar in the bloodstream.

All the starchy foods have some amount of fiber, a non-caloric component of grains and vegetables, which is the roughage of the plant, the plant skeleton. We need to recognize the foods that contain more fiber. There is soluble fiber in fruits, legumes and oats, and insoluble fiber, as in wheat, buckwheat, and vegetables. Chewy things usually have more insoluble fiber. Both fibers are useful.

A high fiber diet is an excellent treatment for bowel regularity, particularly when there is adequate fluid intake and physical activity. A high fiber diet is a treatment for diverticular disease. Soluble fiber found in kidney beans, peas, oats, buckwheat, etc., is shown to improve cholesterol, cardiovascular disease and diabetes control. Choosing unprocessed foods (whole vegetables, unmilled grains, whole fruits) will help ensure an adequate supply of fiber.

Foods rich in fiber slow the digestion of carbohydrates and entry of glucose into the bloodstream, helping the insulin action. Whole grain breads, dried beans, lentils, high fiber breakfast cereals and garden vegetables are important sources of fiber. How would you know that you take enough fiber with your meals? If you have daily easy, large bowel movements (that float!) then you are taking enough fiber. If you do not have any medical reason for constipation (e.g., hypothyroidism) and but are still constipated, then you are probably not eating enough fiber.

Unfortunately, Westernization of societies creates advanced processes for refining foods, depleting the fiber from food plants. Removing the bran and wheat germ from whole-wheat kernels makes white flour. The bran coating of brown rice is removed to produce white rice. Processing this fiber out of your food also removes protein, vitamins and minerals.

The high-fiber diet concept was popularized by Dr Denis Burkitt, who observed that cancer of the colon rarely occurred in populations eating foods with high fiber content. Their diets included a large proportion of fruits and unrefined grains, and the bowel movements tended to be large, bulky, and frequent. Fiber supplements (e.g., psyllium) have been aggressively marketed and fiber in various forms (including sawdust!) has been added to many foods, which are then marketed as "high fiber." How special! Instead of eating an unrefined diet like Burkitt recommended, we are instead refining the fiber and adding it to our refined-grain diet.

The Case for Whole Grains

A major benefit of whole grains is that they contain much more protein and vitamins than their refined counterparts. This is important for several reasons. Protein helps you to feel fed, in contrast with carbohydrates, which can make you feel hungrier. Also, when the protein found in grains is combined with the protein from beans, nuts and seeds, the result is high-quality protein that rivals meat in nutritional value.

Whole grains also contain vitamins, minerals and fiber in the seed coat. The vitamins are useful for the fine metabolic processes of the body. The fiber is useful for helping to slow the absorption of carbohydrate (and the resulting secretion of insulin), as well as keeping your bowels regular. There is ample scientific evidence that high fiber foods have multiple beneficial effects on digestion, regularity, cholesterol levels, and insulin sensitivity.

Certain nutrients found in the seed coat of whole grains are used by our bodies to digest and burn the starch. For example, certain B vitamins and minerals, such as magnesium, are required for breaking down sugar in the cells to produce energy. These vitamins and minerals are available in the seed coat, and help us use the starch contained within the grains. Pretty clever, huh? What happens if the seed coat is removed when the grain is refined and polished? We are left with starch, but no vitamins, and no minerals. Do we still need the vitamins and minerals to metabolize the starch? The answer is yes, but sadly these must come from our body stores, since they've been removed from the food!

The thought of selling a product that depletes our body stores of vitamins and minerals seems pretty strange. How do they get away with it? The answer is simple. Refined grains are easier to store. Insects and other pests tend to leave white flour, white rice and other refined products alone, because they can't survive on them. What does that tell you?

So there you have it: you are now under doctors' orders to use more whole grains in your meals. Whole grains include brown rice, whole wheat, corn, barley, millet, oats, and many other exotic types (amaranth, quinoa). Buckwheat is technically not a grain, but you may treat it like a grain for simplicity. Combine the grains with beans, nuts, seeds, soy and mushrooms for protein and flavor, with vegetables for other nutrients, more fiber, and more flavor.

Just as with meats, a major concern with carbohydrates is the size of the portions. A large bowl of pasta, potatoes or white rice is commonly a part of daily dinner in many families. Toast or bread is an additional source of carbohydrates that are added to the meal, often without any concern about Calories. This is a major reason for weight gain, considering that in many cases the carbohydrates are prepared with some oil or butter or sauces. But it is more complicated than that. Insulin-resistant people will be programmed to convert the high starch meal into fat. Even worse, diabetics may find that even a single slice of bread may cause the blood glucose to rise above 200.

Carbohydrate intake, or we should say the total amount of carbohydrates, is a very important reason for weight gain in many people. Any carbohydrate in the diet stimulates insulin production. More simple carbohydrates and more starches mean more insulin. And, of course, fat helps to double or triple the calories. So, just like with fats, we need to pay attention to the portions. We need to choose high-quality carbohydrates, those with higher protein, vitamin and fiber content. Whenever possible, replace the "white" varieties with the whole grain varieties. There is recent evidence that high carbohydrate diets raise the triglyceride levels more dramatically than high fat diets and play an important role in developing CAD. All the evidence is based on the diets where carbohydrates were refined and westernized. In any case, the portions for starchy meals should be downsized and, as much as possible, substituted with fiber-rich whole grain varieties.

Vegetables sometimes are called free foods because you can eat them without counting the Calories. They are low in Calories, large in volume, and rich in vitamins and nutrients. Vegetables are a wonderful source of fiber. Fresh or cooked, they should be a large part of your everyday menu. Choose seasonal veggies, preferably locally grown. We prefer organically grown produce for its lower pesticide residues and enhanced mineral content.

Vegetables also happen to contain some carbohydrate. For practical purposes, this could be ignored. For instance, if you tried to fatten yourself up by gorging on vegetables, you might actually lose weight, since there would be less room for high-carbohydrate or high-fat foods. Still, too much of anything is not good. Large amounts of cabbage, beets or carrots, for instance, can raise your blood sugar and make you feel bloated.

Fruits are also high in fiber and other nutrients. They are, however, a source of concentrated sugar and may raise blood sugar in susceptible persons. Fresh, unsweetened berries eaten in season tend to have a lower sugar content than sweeter fruits such as peaches and apricots. Use caution with melons and grapes. They are popular throughout the year (thanks to modern transportation methods), but, in fact, are seasonal only in the late summer and autumn. Bananas are popular throughout the year (and have been advertised as the perfect food), but are sugary and probably should be limited. Choosing seasonal and locally-grown fruits would give you higher vitamin content, better taste, stronger local farming economy. When in doubt, diabetics should check blood sugar.

Avoid foods high in simple carbohydrates, like sweetened juices, sodas, candy. These are useless calories that make your pancreas work overtime and wear it out. These will definitely rob your body of vitamins and minerals. Teach your children to avoid simple carbohydrates, explaining to them about the effect on teeth, obesity, etc. Also, please stop stuffing candy in children's party bags. The kid might like it, but his or her pancreas doesn't need the hassle!

Measuring Carbohydrate Servings

If your goal is to lose weight, then you need to do some math. A 1200–1800 Calorie diet will help you lose weight, depending on your gender and physical activity level (for women, 1200–1400 Calories; for men, 1600–1800 Calories).

A crude estimate for the number of Calories you need to eat daily to maintain your weight is your weight in pounds multiplied by 10. For women, the conversion is a little lower, around 9, since women normally tend to have more fat as a percentage of body weight. Thus, Jim, a 170 pound man, burns roughly 1700 Calories per day. If Jim eats only 1200 Calories per day, at the end of one week, he will have eaten roughly 3500 Calories less than he burned, and he will lose approximately 1 pound of fat. We'll do another example with Jim's brother, Joe, later in the book.

Roughly 45% of Calories should come from carbohydrates, which will be about 540–850 Calories or 135–210 grams of carbohydrate daily. One serving of carbohydrates contains about 15 grams of carbohydrates, so your daily servings count would be 9–14 servings per day.

Following are some commonly used starches and fruits transformed into servings. Most of these foods contain protein or fat in addition to carbohydrates, but these are predominantly starchy foods.

If you need to lose weight and are eating 1200 Calories, then you will eat 9 servings of carbohydrates. If 2 starches will be eaten as fruits, 1 as snack, then you can have 2 servings with each of your meals. That is not a lot considering that you are also eating low saturated fat diet. But it is satiating.

It is more important not to eat the unnecessary Calories than to count them, but this rough calculation will help you to manage your portions.

TABLE 6

Carbohydrate Serving Size Equivalents

Food/Quantity	Carbohydrate Servings
Bagel or Muffin–1	2
Bread–1 slice	1
Cereal, cooked–1 cup	2
Cereal, dry unsweetened–$^1/_3$ cup, with milk	2
Pancakes, (4 inch) with syrup–2	2
Pasta, noodles (cooked)–1 cup	2
Potatoes–1 large or 2 small	2
Rice–$^2/_3$ cup	2
Pretzels–15 mini	1
Crackers–10 saltine	1
Tortillas–2 medium	2
Fruit juice, unsweetened–1 cup	2
Fruit, canned–$^1/_2$ cup	1
Corn, beans, lentils–$^1/_2$ cup	1
Apple–1	1
Pear–1	1
Grapes–12–15	1
Melon or Watermelon–1cup	1
Raisins–2 tablespoons	1
Banana–1 large	2

Rules for Carbohydrate, Starch, and Fiber Intake

1. Avoid simple carbohydrates (sweetened juices, sodas, candy).
2. Limit your portions of complex carbohydrates (potatoes, rice, noodles and pasta). Use foods that are high in fiber, including whole grain starches and legumes.

3. Eat lots of salads and vegetables—learn to eat them plain. Use olive oil (or flax oil) with vinegar for dressing.

4. Avoid fatty toppings, sauces, and dressings to limit the Calories.

5. Limit the amount of fruit to 2–3 servings per day. Fruits make excellent snacks and desserts, particularly when they replace donuts, chips, and candy bars between meals.

If you have diabetes and are taking insulin, then you need to know how to precisely calculate your carbohydrates. This information is widely available in the publications on dietary guidelines for diabetics.

Suggested Daily Menus

Now that we have summarized some general ideas for healthy eating, these are some suggestions for easy meal plans. Based on the previous paragraphs, we will try to modify the typical American diet into a healthy diet that is suitable for you and your family.

Version 3 will be a vegetarian choice. Version 5 in all menus can be used for weight loss. It contains minimal amount of carbohydrates. It is a low carbohydrate, low Calorie diet that will help to decrease body weight. Version 6 will be a suggestion for what to choose in the restaurant.

Keep in mind that Europeans tend to eat their largest meal at midday and a lighter evening meal. This makes good sense, given that we are most active during the day, and won't reflux so much at night if we eat a light evening meal.

BREAKFAST

Version 1

1 bowl whole grain cereal with low fat milk, with 10–12 raisins or dried cranberries. Add 1–2 tablespoons sunflower seeds or 3–4 walnuts to boost protein and flavor. Drink a cup of hot tea or coffee, instead of juice.

Version 2

Two slices whole-wheat toast, with yogurt topping or cheese, or 1–2 boiled eggs. My Auntie recommends Lebni, a form of yogurt with the water drained out, over the bread with a little olive oil on top! See if you can find zaatar (thyme and herb mixture) in a Middle Eastern market to sprinkle over the top.

Version 3 (Vegetarian)

$^1/_2$ or 1 cup hot cereal, with water or soy milk, with 1 teaspoon of brown sugar or honey. Again, throw in some sunflower seeds or sliced almonds for flavor.

Version 4

$^1/_2$ whole-wheat bagel with low fat cream cheese spread or lox. Add half a dozen almonds that have soaked in water overnight.

Version 5 (Weight loss)

3–4 tablespoons of cottage cheese with a tangerine or half a pear.

Version 6 (Restaurant)

You may have an omelet or ham. A veggie (onions, mushroom, and peppers) omelet is an excellent fancy, healthy breakfast served with whole-wheat pocket bread. Avoid sausages, bacon and "combo plates." You will still enjoy your breakfast and stop thinking after breakfast, "I ate too much." Ask for hot tea or coffee instead of orange juice.

Version 7

Brown rice and vegetables left over from the night before. You can quickly reheat the food by spilling a bit of boiling water on top.

Version 8 (Vegetarian)

Tofu scramble: quickly made by sautéing onions and mushrooms in a little olive oil. When moderately cooked, place a 3–4 ounce slab of tofu on top. As it warms up, mash it coarsely with a fork. Dust it with a little turmeric for a nice yellow color, season with salt and pepper. It will look and taste like scrambled eggs. Enjoy with a slice of whole grain toast and a cup of tea or coffee.

Drinks: coffee, tea, milk, or $1/2$ cup unsweetened juices. Avoid sugar or high fat creamer.

LUNCH

Version 1

Soup and salad (from your cafeteria is good, however, the crackers served usually contain partially hydrogenated oils and the dressing sometimes is already premixed). Make your own dressing with olive oil and vinegar, avoid the crackers and, instead, have a slice of whole wheat bread, with or without butter.

Version 2

Sandwich and a fruit is an excellent lunch. (Pre-made sandwiches usually have too much mayo and too much meat.) Make your own sandwich on whole wheat bread, a thin layer of mustard or butter, one slice of cold cuts and cheese, and lettuce, pickles (if you do not have high blood pressure) and tomatoes as you wish. Stuffed pita bread, tacos and burritos are great for lunch or dinner.

How do you make a sandwich? Do you add enough meat to wash down the whole grain bread? Or do you add enough bread to the meat to keep your fingers from becoming greasy?

Version 3 (Vegetarian)

Veggie burger or soyburger and salad or fruit (instead of French fries).

Version 4 (Dr Jerry's favorite)

Brown rice about half full in a deep bowl. Top generously with cooked beans or tofu. Adorn with chopped nuts, pumpkin seeds, or nut butter. Fill the bowl with vegetable leftovers from last night (or steamed this morning!) Add $1/2$ tsp of finely chopped pickles. Pour a little hemp seed oil over the top and garnish with plum vinegar or a drop of soy sauce. Cover with a small plate and take it to work!

Version #5 (Weight loss)

Soup and salad. Add beans, tofu, mushrooms, artichoke hearts and sunflower seeds from the salad bar. Skip the crackers and go easy on the bread.

Version #6 (Restaurant)

Pass on the fries, salad dressing, bread and butter, mayo and sodas and you will cut down on a lot of unneeded calories. Whatever you do beyond this should be okay.

Drinks: Calistoga drink, hot tea, iced tea, tomato juice or a shake with non-fat milk and fruit.

Snacks: 2–3 whole-wheat crackers, baby carrots, celery sticks, fresh peppers, low fat popcorn, low fat yogurt, and fruit. A handful of almonds or sunflower seeds is filling. Make sure you are having no more than one serving at a time. For children, cheese stick, yogurt or a peanut butter and jelly sandwich are a great alternatives for Oreos or chips.

DINNER

Include all food groups in your dinner. If you try to go meatless (great idea), then carefully consider your protein sources. Use beans, lentils, nuts and seeds freely. These can also supplement animal-based proteins (e.g., trout amandine). Serve a large salad with meals, eat the salad plain or use vinaigrette dressing. Add walnut halves, hazelnuts or sunflower seeds to the salad.

Use the palm of your hand (not including fingers) as a measure for the size of meats (red, chicken or fish). Choose lean cuts of meat, loin and round cuts of beef, loin and leg cuts for pork and lamb. Choose cooking methods that require little fat, such as baking, steaming, broiling, grilling and roasting. Remove skin and visible fat from meat before serving.

High fiber whole grain starches are preferable. Use brown rice, bulgur, millet, buckwheat, or pasta (no more than $^1/_2$ to $^3/_4$ cup) as an addition to the meal. Use olive oil as your main cooking oil.

You can steam or sauté any veggies and cover the rest of your plate (mushrooms, broccoli, carrots, cabbage, zucchini, green beans, beets, eggplant, cauliflower, spinach, Swiss chard).

Eat slowly and chew your food well. Rethink the need for second helpings of meats or starches.

Drinks: 1–2 glasses of water, wine, mineral water or low fat milk. It's best to drink the water half an hour or so prior to the meal.

Dessert: Pass on it or have fruit. Greatly limit portion size if served pastry.

Version 1

Soup or salad prior to pasta entree will help you minimize the size of the pasta portion. Use a little cheese, mozzarella or Parmesan over the pasta. Soup or salad will substitute well if you are planning to eat pizza for dinner. Avoid pepperoni pizza and too much cheese on any type of pizza. Actually forget the pizza. Proceed to version 2. (A fabulously delicious alternative is vegetarian pizza combo, made without cheese, with anchovies. It usually draws a weird stare from the guy behind the pizza counter. Too bad the pizza joints don't typically use whole-wheat crust.)

Version 2

Large salad of your choice. 3–5 oz lean meat, broiled, baked, barbecued or roasted, and 3 tablespoons of brown rice and steamed vegetables. Or, as a substitute for the rice, a cob of corn without butter.

Version 3 (Vegetarian)

Bowl of barley soup and stir-fry veggies with Boca chicken breast (yummy chicken made of soy), or tofu stuffed into 2 pita bread halves.

Version 4

Bowl of miso soup (you usually have it in Japanese restaurants), about 3 oz broiled or baked fish, $1/2$ cup of wild rice, steamed asparagus and broccoli. Fruit for dessert (1 cup of berries, a slice of watermelon or cantaloupe).

Version 5 (Weight loss)

Large bowl of salad without dressing (use salt and pepper or lemon juice for flavor). 3–5 oz of meat, fish or tofu; collard greens or any other green vegetables, sautéed or steamed, to cover the plate. 2 or 3 tablespoons of lentils, garbanzo beans or kidney beans, from a can or home cooked.

Version 6 (Restaurant)

When you are eating in a restaurant, the first thing to remember is that people tend to eat too much. Pass on hors d'oeuvres and dessert and you will also save some money. In Asian restaurants, you need to watch the amount of carbohydrates, rather than having the 3rd or 4th serving of rice. Avoid deep fried foods in Chinese and Japanese restaurants. In Italian restaurants, the problem is usually the overabundance of pasta. In American restaurants, servings usually include too much meat and fat. Mexican restaurants will overfeed you with corn chips and cheese.

Start with a salad dressed with vinaigrette. 3–5 oz of any lean meat or fish with sautéed vegetables of your choice and green salad. Have non-fat yogurt or fruit for dessert.

Remember that everybody wants you to eat more (including your mom). You are your only advocate!

Version 7

If you like stuffed vegetables, "dolmas" (zucchini, cabbage, tomatoes, grape leaves, etc.), you may use bulgur or brown rice, instead of white rice, to mix with ground meat.

Bon Appetite!

Once you have changed your diet and eat like this, you will be consuming about 1200–2000 Calories/day. Closer to 1200 Calories you will lose weight, and closer to 1800–2000 Calories/day you will maintain your weight. You should eat like this on 9 out of 10 days. What about that one day? Well, once in a while you can have junk food, but you know what? With time, it will taste too rich, greasy and heavy. Used in moderation and selectively, you won't be harmed.

Moderation is like a sunken treasure lost in the oversized race of everyday objectives: working too much, eating too much, drinking or smoking too much. Let us raise the treasure of moderation and share it among ourselves. We will then enjoy our food and health for many years to come.

11

Exercise to Fit Your Daily Schedule

Attention to health is Life's greatest hindrance.

—Plato

What is the sound of exercise? Grunt. Sweat. Lift. Press. Buns of steel. Thirty miles per week. Forty-five minutes on the Stairmaster. But I haven't kept it up for the past three months. I'm always walking (at work).

Let's face it. Life in the United States is sedentary. We watch TV, sit too long at the computer, drive places where we could have walked or biked, and spend another ninety seconds in the parking lot looking for a parking space closer to the Pizza Parlor door. We prefer escalators and elevators to the stairs. We sat at the computer to write this book and you are sitting in a couch or chair reading it. (If you happen to be reading this while exercising, e-mail us at once and we'll use you as a poster-child for the next edition!) Sedentary life is one of the two dragon heads creating the epidemics of obesity in this country. Your guess is right. The other one is unhealthy food, the main player in the previous chapter.

Sedentarism (we made up a new word) is a social disease that starts from early childhood, when we start to let our children watch too many video cartoons, then video games, then computer games. It is a disease of the late twentieth century that we are boldly taking with us to the next millennium. Sedentarism is the major environmental factor for obesity and insulin resistance.

Whatever its sound, exercise is part of a healthy lifestyle and part of the treatment of Metabolic Syndrome. Exercise has shown its value in many ways that do not necessarily follow the same line of thinking.

The Benefits of Exercise

Function begets function. This is good advice to the elderly, the infirm, the unstable. A 65 year old (whether insulin resistant or not) who exercises is, on average, going to be more mobile and secure on his feet. This is important when one considers the number of broken hips due to falls, an injury carrying up to a 20% mortality rate! Among diabetics aged 55 or older, over half reported *zero* minutes of weekly physical activity. Hello?!? Among these patients, there was belief that exercise should be curtailed in the elderly, and should be avoided in persons with high blood pressure (both untrue).

Improves hypertension. The effect of exercise to improve mild-to-moderate hypertension is again independent of weight loss. Decrease in both systolic and diastolic blood pressures (upper and lower numbers of blood pressure) of 5–10 mmHg are common and are often correlated with decreases in serum insulin and triglyceride levels. Ample studies showed exercise improves cardiovascular function, increases fitness and physical working capacity, and improves sense of well being and quality of life.

People with Metabolic Syndrome or diabetes should be screened for cardiac disease before starting a vigorous exercise program. Visit your doctor and discuss it. Evaluation may include an electrocardiogram or a treadmill test, because it is important to determine whether you already have heart disease before putting a heavy workload on your cardiovascular system.

Affects body weight. Even if the weight stays the same, some fat is exchanged for muscle during exercise. How many of our patients have stated that their weight remained unchanged while on an exercise program, but their clothes fit better. It is clear that exercise leads to a shift in body weight. Some of the fat is replaced by muscle, which is more dense than fat. Interestingly, in insulin-resistant patients, exercise leads to preferential removal of fat from the abdominal cavity; this is presumably related to its beneficial effect on insulin sensitivity.

It is hard to achieve weight loss without exercise. Among obese insulin-resistant patients placed in a lifestyle-change program, a 4.5 kilogram (almost 10 pounds) drop in weight was associated with improved insulin resistance, lowered blood pressure, and reduced risk of developing diabetes.

The effect of exercise on weight loss is additive to that of Calorie restriction. Each pound of fat contains enough food energy to propel a human about 37 miles on foot. It will be difficult, at best, to exercise off all of the pounds we're carrying, but watch what happens when exercise is combined with diet.

Let's do some quick math. Joe weighs 220 lbs. At 10 Calories/lb/day, he is consuming (and burning) 2200 Calories to maintain his weight. If he wants to lose one pound per week, he must burn approximately 3500 Calories more than he eats each week, roughly 500 Calories per day. This will work for a while, but Joe will soon find out that after a few weeks his metabolism will slow, and he will burn fewer Calories to maintain his weight. Let's assume that Joe cuts his food intake to 1700 Calories and after several weeks his metabolic level has dropped to 2000 Calories. He is no longer burning 500 Calories more than he is eating and his weight loss will slow. However, if he runs for a half hour each day, he will burn an extra 200 Calories and make up for the decrease in his metabolic rate.

Weight loss is more complex than this—it is as complex as the individual trying to lose weight. For example, if Joe tries to cut back on Calories by skipping breakfast, his metabolic rate will slow and he will burn up energy more slowly. So, Joe grabs a bowl of oats with a handful of sunflower seeds to tide him over until lunch. Good job, Joe!

Improves self-esteem. Regular exercise improves self-esteem and has an antidepressant effect. Physical training benefits the psychological response to stress. In other words, a healthy mind needs a healthy body. In any case, you will be amazed how quickly a depressed mood improves after vigorous activity.

Improves insulin resistance. Exercise has been shown to improve insulin resistance and glucose tolerance independent of its effect on weight. This means that even if your weight remains constant, you can enjoy some of the positive health benefits shared by your thin-as-a-rail neighbor who jogged by your house at five o'clock this morning.

Important for diabetics. Exercise is an important component of treatment of all people with diabetes. It lowers the blood glucose concentration during and after exercise. It lowers insulin concentration and improves insulin action. It improves Hemoglobin A_{1C}, the measure of chronic blood sugar control.

If you are on treatment for diabetes (either pills or insulin injections), you are able to exercise, but you must pay careful attention to your blood sugar. Certain medications for diabetes can cause low blood sugar (hypoglycemia). This is true whether or not you exercise, but if you exercise on some days and not on others, your blood sugar might drop too low on the days when you do work out. After all, the medication is just a pill (or injection), and the medication has no way of knowing what you've eaten, or how much you are going to exercise. Work closely with your physician.

Obese patients put on a diet dropped insulin levels by 22%, compared with patients put on a diet plus an aerobic exercise program who dropped their levels by 40%. This is quite significant. Insulin resistant people have circulating insulin levels that are roughly double what is normal. A 40 percent drop translates to near normalization of insulin levels.

Improves lipid profile. Another benefit from exercise is the improvement of the lipid profile. Physical training is associated with a significant decrease in serum triglycerides, slight reduction of LDL-C and increase of HDL-C. This is exactly what you need; however, the improvement in the lipid profile requires an exercise program of fairly high intensity. Improvement in the lipid profile is observed with running >9 miles a week, and increases progressively up to 40 miles a week. This level of training is not realistic for many of our patients. So, it makes sense to combine exercise with diet, adding medications if necessary.

Prolongs life. This is reminiscent of the story of the man who gave up smoking, drinking and womanizing. He didn't live a hundred years, but it sure seemed like it. In one study, however, subjects who exercised had improved immune function as measured by fewer colds and fewer sick days from work. In any case, given that heart attacks and cardiovascular disease are the leading killers (by far) of people in the United States, it makes good sense to exercise if you plan to be around for a while.

What is the Best Exercise?

The best exercise is something you enjoy doing. This makes sense. What is the point of running miles and miles if all the weight is going to return as soon as you stop? More than that, what is the point if you are going to lose all of the other health benefits after you stop exercising? In one study, all of the health benefits, including the effects on insulin resistance, glycemic control and blood pressure control, were lost within four months after stopping exercise. Compliance with the exercise program and changes of lifestyle are important habits. Easy to start, hard to continue. "I am tired today," "It is raining," "There is no time," and many others.

Here are several suggestions. Choose a program that you enjoy, use a variety of exercise routines that can be substituted, and make an exercise out of non-exercise activity. For instance walk faster at work, never take an elevator or escalator, park your car as far as possible from your destination and always return the shopping cart. Take a bicycle to the market. Do not be lazy; do not be afraid of being inefficient. Don't worry about being late. The payoff of your exercise program is fewer visits to the doctor, fewer days in the hospital! Walking is an excellent exercise, since it is also a convenient means of transportation. Walking is our own exercise of choice. People who walk 1.5 miles daily have $^1/_2$ of the risk of mortality compared to people who do not walk at all. Brisk walking gives you even more cardiovascular benefit. In your case, your preference may be different. The important thing is that you keep it up and don't give up after a few weeks. What do you like to do? Bicycling is even more convenient than walking as a means of transportation. Both bicycling and walking can be combined with buses or trains. Running is wonderful for breaking a sweat and getting that endorphin rush. Gardening is a good way to exercise the upper extremities and trunk muscles, the beauty ultimately reflected in your physique, as well as in your garden.

Hiking is a great way of spending time with family and friends. Swimming, tennis, Ping-Pong, volleyball, dancing, aerobics, jazzercise, Curves®, golf, karate, weight lifting, walking on a treadmill while watching TV, walking in a mall on a rainy day—everything works, just do it— every day.

Anything is better than nothing! If your goal is weight reduction, then you need to exercise at least 5 days a week (and eat a healthy diet 7 days a week). If your goal is improving your blood sugar or cardiovascular condition, then you need to exercise at least 3 days a week (and eat a healthy diet 7 days a week). As noted earlier, it has been shown that to improve the lipid profile, you need to do more vigorous exercise than for blood glucose control or fitness.

If you are older than 55, exercise should be an important part of your lifestyle. It helps with balance, increases strength and flexibility. No matter what medications you take to prevent osteoporosis, exercise should accompany the treatment of osteoporosis. The mere act of putting your old bones to work causes them to more effectively hold on to calcium. People who are immobilized for any reason have a rapid bone loss. Less toned/trained people are prone to falls, a major problem in elderly population.

Be Realistic

Choose an exercise program that fits your daily schedule. Start slowly, build up gradually. Remember, exercise is safe and has no side effects if it is used correctly. Do not start jogging if the last time you jogged was 10 years ago. We have all heard the stories of people who have died from a heart attack while running.

Listen to your body as you increase your exercise volume and intensity. Unusual chest pains, an inappropriately accelerated heart rate, shortness of breath, etc., should alert one to consult his or her physician.

Start out slowly and use your head. Horace said, "Be fond of what you are and what you can do and not what you would like to be or to do."

12

Alcohol and Smoking

When we are conquered by the strength of wine
Our limbs grow heavy, our legs intertwine;
With sodden mind, slow tongue, and swimming eyes
We reel amid hiccups, brawls and cries.

—Lucretius

This is a vivid description of drunkenness. Heavy drinking is defined as a quantity of alcohol consumption that exceeds an established threshold value. The National Institute of Alcohol Abuse and Alcoholism sets this threshold at more than 14 drinks per week for men (or >4 drinks per occasion); and more than 7 drinks per week for women (or >3 drinks on occasion). 1 drink is considered 12 ounces (355 ml) of beer, a 4 ounce (118 ml) glass of wine or a 1.5 ounce (44 ml) shot of liquor.

Recently, there is more and more evidence on reduced CAD and all-cause mortality in light-to-moderate drinkers. The benefit of alcohol seems greatest in certain individuals, such as people with diabetes who are at higher risk of cardiovascular diseases. It was also shown that people who drink 1–2 glasses of wine daily have lower risk of developing diabetes, when compared with nondrinkers or those drinking more than 2 drinks per day.

The proposed mechanisms for this include the anti-atherogenic effect of alcohol due to elevation of HDL-C, decreased clotting, and improvement of insulin resistance. Alcohol, by the way, is a fourth form of Calories, in addition to fat, protein and carbohydrate. Alcohol contains 7 Calories per gram, compared with 4 for protein and carbohydrate, and 9 for fat. As with fats, alcohol does not require the action of insulin in order to be used as fuel.

Excess alcohol is not heart healthy. More than 2 drinks per day can raise blood pressure, depress the immune system, and damage the liver, pancreas, and nervous system.

Smoking is bad for you. Everybody knows that. There are at least fifteen common diseases that are caused or worsened by smoking, and even more minor diseases that are aggravated by it. The data shows pretty clearly that smokers tend to not live as long as non-smokers. In fact, it is so obviously a bad habit that we are not going to waste time any more with anti-smoking hype. Decreased rates of smoking, along with the better diagnosis and treatment of high blood pressure and cholesterol, are the likely causes of some decline in cardiovascular mortality in this country.

Regarding insulin resistance, there is data that smoking decreases insulin sensitivity. At the same time, smoking decreases appetite, and many people notice mild-to-moderate weight gain after smoking cessation.

A former first lady, clarifying why a cigarette tax was proposed to fund health care, explained that cigarettes were the only product which, when used as directed, kill. It makes a good slogan, but the same could be said for whipped cream, margarine, and fast food chains.

13

Complementary and Alternative Management

Life is not merely being alive, but being well.
—Martial, Epigrams

Primary goals are still weight loss and exercise. But read on. . . . There is not much scientific evidence supporting alternative treatments. Your local Farmers' Market has not been able to sponsor any studies, nor has your local health food store. Much of the information in this chapter is based on the publications of "The Lawrence Review of Natural Products" and is based on European studies.

Supplements

When you are considering making lifestyle changes, most of these suggestions are pertinent recommendations for everyday life. Following are some of the foods, minerals, vitamins and herbal preparations that are known to be beneficial in glucose metabolism and atherosclerosis. It is not surprising that some of those concomitantly improve cholesterol profiles and have lured more interest and scientific research than others. We will review them from the standpoint of possible mechanism of action, efficacy, benefits, and safety issues. There is much more out there on the market, but these are the ones worth discussing.

Dietary fiber is one the most important supplements you should use. Psyllium seed husks are commonly used as commercial bulk laxatives.

This product works by swelling up with water, and it should be taken with large amount of fluids. It is not absorbed by the gut. Psyllium was shown to lower cholesterol and improve the glucose control in diabetics. The main side effect is bloating and flatulence. It can decrease the absorption of some drugs (so don't take it at the same time as prescribed medication); also note that allergy to psyllium is reported. If you are not consuming enough fiber from foods, you should consider adding psyllium to your diet, usually 1–2 tablespoons daily. It is marketed as Metamucil or Konsyl and others. We recommend the use of psyllium as a temporary fix while you are making the transition to a high-fiber diet; but certain patients, such as the fast-food addict with diverticulosis, may require psyllium for the long term.

Guar gum is similar to psyllium, in that it forms a mucilaginous mass in the intestines. It regulates glucose metabolism by slowing down glucose absorption. It improves cholesterol and blood pressure. The recommended dose is 3 grams (about $1/_2$ teaspoon) three times daily. It is not absorbed, needs to be taken with a large amount of water, and may interfere with absorption of drugs by binding to them in the gut.

Buckwheat usage in diabetics is popular in Eastern Europe. The likely mechanism is the high fiber content and slow absorption of glucose. It is delicious and safe to use when cooked or soaked in milk or yogurt. It has no side effects. Buckwheat is 14% protein by dry weight. It is gluten-free and useful for those who cannot eat wheat.

Garlic is the most well known food-plant with numerous beneficial effects; the ancient Egyptians knew of its virtues. There is strong evidence demonstrating its beneficial effect on the cholesterol pattern, and some weak evidence for improving glucose metabolism. Many other possible benefits are antioxidant effects, decreased blood clotting, mild improvement of blood pressure, antiseptic, antibacterial, and antifungal activity, and improving immunity. There are no side effects, except for the smell. How much should one take? As much fresh garlic as you can. Mince or grind your garlic well; air exposure seems to activate its beneficial chemicals. Dosage is somewhat arbitrary for commercial preparations and there is considerable variability in their effect.

Fenugreek spice is commonly sold as a dried ripe seed and is used as a spice. It improves cholesterol and blood sugar levels in hyperlipidemic and diabetic people. Mostly, it lowers triglyceride level. The seeds are rich in fiber, which may be the main reason it can lower blood sugar levels. Seeds have a bitter taste and encapsulated products are available. Recommended usage is 5–30 grams with each meal or 15–60 grams with one meal, once daily. Intestinal upset and nausea can occur with doses of more than 100 grams. Fresh fenugreek herb is sometimes used.

Siberian Ginseng or Eleutheroccocus is commonly used in Russia and China. A decrease in plasma glucose was shown in both animal and human studies; the mechanism is unknown. Adaptogenic and immune-boosting properties are also described. With high doses of more than 1 gram daily, excitation of the nervous system is reported.

Essential fatty acids (EFAs, omega-3 and omega-6 fatty acids) are certain fatty acids that are not made by the body and should be eaten with our foods to maintain the normal metabolism. (See our discussion on Fat consumption, Chapter 10.) EFAs are shown to decrease blood pressure, improve the cardiovascular profile, decrease clotting, decrease inflammation and lower cholesterol by lowering triglycerides.

Omega-3 fatty acids are found in fish oil, and deep cold water fish (like salmon, herring, sardines and tuna). Docosahexaenoic acid (DHA) and Eicosapentoic acid (EPA) are two omega-3 fatty acids that are shown to trim the cardiovascular risk. When compared with olive oil, 4 grams of DHA was more protective of cardiac risk. The amount of omega-3 varies with fish species and geography. Fish themselves obtain the omega-3 fatty acids from plankton, so the colder the water, the higher the omega-3 of the fish that live in it. 100 grams of Atlantic salmon daily contains enough DHA to supply the recommended amount. The other rich source for 3-omega fatty acids is flaxseed oil. Numerous positive effects are demonstrated in people using flaxseed oil, including improved cholesterol patterns, cardiovascular benefit and anti-inflammatory effect. Both fish oil and flax oil are available in health food stores in liquid form as well as in capsule form.

The role of vitamins is becoming unclear. Much of the food that we are consuming was picked from the fields a long time ago, or else it is processed and refined. All these factors deplete the vitamins. If you are not doing your own gardening and do not have regular access to a Farmer's Market, then consider taking a daily multivitamin. However, the evidence for antioxidants, in particular vitamin C and vitamin E, is conflicting. Originally, they were considered beneficial for heart disease prevention. Recent evidence, however, has shown them to negate the beneficial effect of a commonly used (and expensive) cholesterol-lowering drug.

Other antioxidants include selenium, lipoic acid, anthocyanins, olive leaf extract, and others. While these may be beneficial, one might also suppose that eliminating oxidants from our environment (animal products, cigarette smoke, automobile exhaust, chlorinated water—have I hit a nerve yet?) will achieve the same end.

Some of the vitamins have been shown to be of more importance in insulin resistant people and diabetics, who have a tendency to cardiovascular disease. Nicotinic acid (niacin) improves some of the cardiac risk factors (increases HDL and decreases triglycerides), and is available in prescription and OTC forms; however, it is hard to tolerate and it may cause mild deterioration of glucose tolerance. Folic acid is also used in certain patients with high homocysteine levels; and vitamin B complex is often advised for patients taking folic acid.

Vanadium or vanadyl sulfate is a trace mineral with demonstrated insulin-sensitizing effect. In animal studies, it was shown to decrease insulin levels in the blood and improve glucose utilization by the muscle and liver. It is not well understood how it works, but there is scientific evidence that it improves insulin action, lowers blood glucose and hemoglobin A_{1C}. Human studies done with a daily intake of 50–150 mg showed an improved glucose metabolism that lasted for some time, even after the mineral was discontinued. At the beginning, it can cause some gastrointestinal upset that resolves soon after. It is unclear how vanadium is excreted from the body, but no real toxicity has been reported so far. There are no long term studies done with vanadyl sulfate, so the usage at this point can be recommended for short periods of time (4–6 weeks).

Chromium picolinate is shown to improve insulin resistance, blood sugar, cholesterol profile and hemoglobin A_{1c}. It has been demonstrated to improve the body composition by increasing muscle mass and, possibly, causing mild weight loss. Chromium is identified as the Glucose Tolerance Factor of yeast, and many chromium supplements use the term GTF. Government surveys suggest that most Americans fail to get even 50 micrograms of chromium per day. Foods that are rich in chromium are string beans, whole grains, eggs, cucumber, soy foods, organ meats, onions, garlic, fruits, shiitake mushroom and wheat germ. The recommended amount is 200–400 mcg in two divided doses. There is some evidence that chromium picolinate diminishes carbohydrate craving. Most of the OTC weight loss drugs contain chromium as one of the important ingredients.

Ethnobotanical literature lists dozens of herbs used worldwide to treat diabetes. These uses are handed down from generation to generation. Standardization is difficult, because the active chemical content of plants may vary from batch to batch. A number of these are common spices, including garlic and fenugreek, which are mentioned above. Others, including Stevia, are not used directly to lower blood sugar, but as part of a lifestyle change, by helping to eliminate sugar from the diet.

Stevia is an herb that has been used worldwide as a sweetener. It is 20–30 times sweeter than sugar, but contains a negligible amount of Calories and does not raise blood sugar. It is sold either as the raw herb, the powdered herb, or as an extract. The herb itself has a slightly grassy aftertaste that may be distracting. Importation of Stevia was temporarily banned by the Food and Drug Administration over many voiced protests because of confusion as to whether it was a food or a drug (greatly simplified statement). Anyway, the ban has been lifted and you will see the use of Stevia increasing during the next few years.

Another herb to mention here is licorice. Licorice root contains compounds that are, like Stevia, many times sweeter than sugar and may be used to add a sweet taste to other foods. Overuse of licorice may raise blood pressure.

Complementary Living

I have a fantasy about opening a market. In the *Food* section, there are whole grains, fresh produce, fresh meats, nuts, and teas. You know, fresh. In the *"Food"* section (the sign on the wall over this area contains the quotation marks) are the canned and frozen vegetables, the processed meats, the white bread and polished grains. There is also a *Not Really Food* section containing the soft drinks, the potato chips, mayonnaise, and a number of other products where the processing and packaging is out of proportion to the ingredients that went into them. My customers would ask about the difference between *Food* and *"Food"* (answer me that, and you will know all of medicine). They would chuckle as they sneak a few items out of the *Not Really Food* section. They might not even notice that I did most of my own shopping at the health food store around the block.

Let's make a few things clear. Eating is not a science. If it were, it would need to be studied in the context of the question "Who am I?" Go back to the last paragraph and read it again. Can you imagine confronting customers with the difference between *Food* and *"Food"*? Can you imagine challenging them to wander into the *Not Really Food* section to grab a candy bar?

Who am I, anyway? In the 1960s there was the Hippie movement, flower children dropping out of life to "figure out who I am." It was amusing. It was all so, so counter-culture. In reality, it is vital. "Who I am" determines everything. It determines how I dress, how I drive a car, what I eat, whether I smoke, whether I yell at the kids, how I respond to advertisement. In many respects, who I am determines who you are.

Many patients we see and treat in our office have problems related to diet and obesity. We discuss diet with our patients on a regular basis. It would be nice to use other words besides "diet," since that word implies that we are going to "put the patient on a diet." Being put on a diet is often construed by the patient as punitive.

Who am I, anyway? The doctor just asked me about diet. Am I on a good diet or a bad diet? Will the doctor yell at me? Will I have to stand in the corner? I really am a failure. Why is the doctor being so mean to me, anyway? No wonder my blood pressure is so high.

Is a car good or bad? Is a piece of chicken good or bad? Is a candy bar good or bad? They're neither. They are just a car, a piece of chicken, a candy bar. Is an obese hypertensive diabetic who likes to eat fast food good or bad? The answer to that question has to do with this whole "Who am I?" issue. Anyway, we love everybody and are not going to send that person to stand in the corner. So let's forget good and bad. Let's move on. On to "Who am I?" On to "What do I want?" On to "What's for dinner?"

In college I was accustomed to a well rounded diet: chuck steak, French bread, a head of lettuce, and a can of beer. It contained three of the four basic food groups (omitting dairy, but I could have milk on my cereal the next morning). I knew that the steak would provide much needed protein and was familiar with the photos of children with kwashiorkor, a condition of protein deficiency.

That was over twenty years ago. Ahh, so much has changed. Fish and chicken. Whole wheat bread. Broccoli and spinach. Bottled beer.

Vegetarianism and macrobiotics make diet one of the quintessential "alternative" treatments because they provide so many choices to answer the question, "What's for dinner?"

Let me quote Jake, a patient who refused surgical treatment for severe blockage of the carotid arteries. My response was to start him on a lipid-lowering drug and tell him, "Congratulations, you are now a vegetarian." His comment, some weeks later, was delightful and startling: "I had no idea there was so much food out there." That is really the essence, the soul of this discussion. Once you understand Jake's comment, you can skip this entire chapter. Once you live Jake's comment, you can put away this entire book.

The term "macrobiotics" refers to the art of prolonging life through healthy and natural life and diet choices. The macrobiotic diet consists roughly of 50% whole grain, 25% vegetables, 10% beans, and smaller quantities of fruits, nuts, soups and animal products. You are encouraged to buy a book on macrobiotics (and read it).

Stress Management

Stress management is a critical piece of the "stay healthy" puzzle. Stress and disease are intertwined like this (I am holding my clasped fingers, can you see?). Healthy people get sick and sick people get sicker when faced with emotional trauma. Probably half of those walking into our waiting room in our busy office are suffering stress-related conditions.

This is not a new idea. Stress scales are standard reading for medical students. A famous paper by Holmes and Rahe assigns higher stress scores for major traumatic life events (such as the death of a spouse or child) and lower stress scores for more mundane hassles, like being fired from a job or being handed a speeding ticket. Scoring high on this stress scale, i.e., having more than a certain aggregate number of stress points, corre-lated quite significantly with risk of hospitalization within the following two years.

There are many ways of expressing the obvious. When a person is exposed to physical or emotional hardship, his/her resistance to disease declines. Thus, the flu that you caught on the airline had more to do with travel fatigue than with the plane's air circulation. The man devel-oped shingles while putting his house up for sale. Chronic stress is asso-ciated with elevations in cortisone production by the adrenal glands. (Keep that freshly in mind, as the cortisone can raise your blood sugar!) And chronic stress often leads to overuse of alcohol and prescription seda-tives, not to mention overeating.

A study in Finland during the cold war identified proximity to the Russian border (and subsequent threat of invasion) as the most signifi-cant predictor of sudden cardiac death. Similar risk was identified in young (otherwise healthy) engineers in the aerospace industry in the United States. These engineers were at constant risk of losing their jobs due to layoffs dictated by the whims of the space race.

Here on the home front, the boss is a jerk. The relationship is on the rocks. We manage our daily hassles of traffic jams, flight delays, stock market corrections, noisy kids. Can you imagine that we need to have the terms "road rage" and "air rage?"

Stress management courses are a booming business, with many satisfied customers. Check it out. We can't replace a weekend course with a chapter in a book. Choose from mindfulness meditation, Tai Chi, transcendental meditation, or an afternoon in church. Meanwhile, there are some basic areas to examine in your own life today.

Are you spending any quiet time alone? With the TV turned off (better yet, unplugged and in the garage)? Have you got a comfortable place to sit outside listening to crickets?

Are you getting out to the local parks and breathing in the fresh air and aroma of the leaves? Are you noticing the graceful sine wave of the squirrel's body and tail?

Are you finding alternatives to fighting traffic? Public transportation allows you to sit, close your eyes, read, or snooze instead of focusing between the rear view mirror and the bumper ahead of you. Walking to a bus stop or train station may well be the only exercise you get today, and public transportation allows you to not be in a hurry for a few precious minutes. (Have you ever tried to be in a hurry while riding the bus?)

We all know the adage to stop and smell the roses—are you actually doing it? Do you stop to admire paintings? Have you tried giving up coffee for two weeks? Have you tried fasting for a day? There is a terrific book, *Be Happier Starting Now,* written by Dr Ray Sahelian, available for about ten bucks. In it, he describes many ideas for spending your time, such as renting a classic old movie or going to a museum. Dr Ray emphasizes these techniques to help increase one's breadth and personal growth—but they have the added bonus of letting you stop and do something besides worry.

Deal with your addictions. Food? Alcohol? Tobacco? Exercise? Romance? Cars? Cards? Coffee? Gossip? TV?

Identify your addiction(s). Come on, there is something. Perhaps it stems from our image of ourselves. What is it in our lives that we can't imagine ourselves without? Imagine the blank stare of patients at the suggestion of giving up fast food or diet soda. Addictions are fed by stress.

The more stressed you are, the more prone you are for going to your addiction of choice. As endless is the list of addictions, the top one is the food: chips, candy, cookies, sodas, coffee, cakes, burgers. The refrigerator is the common place to turn when you are stressed. It used to be the cigarettes, but the antismoking campaign worked. Do we need an antifood campaign? Well, maybe at least stop the fast food juicy ads on TV. We need a better understanding of the harm that you can sustain from unhealthy food. Your health and your life are in your hands; we should not have gotten to the point that we witnessed a lawsuit against fast food chains. Hello! It is your health, and as juicy and cheap as the burger is, it is a danger to your health . . . just like smoking. And just like the occasional cigarette is not going to cause lung cancer, the occasional fast food is unlikely to kill you this year. How do you define "occasional?"

Sometimes we wear our addictions like a badge. "I have a panic disorder so I need my Valium refilled." "I need my Diet Pepsi every day," (an acutely ill anorexic woman actually told me this as a reason why she would keep Diet Pepsi in her hospital room).

Denial is the most powerful force in the entire Universe. It allows diabetics to eat a bag of potato chips and respiratory therapists to smoke a pack of cigarettes per day.

Sometimes our addictions masquerade as lifestyle traps. Consider the diabetic who cannot eat properly because of 16-hour workdays. What advice can we give this poor soul? Is he addicted to fast food? To long work hours? Or is he addicted to the notion that one must put up with this stressful life routine for some greater good?

A good way to deal with an addiction is to replace it with a healthy passion. Try new things: a new class, a new language, walks through new cities; or old favorites: gardening, a forgotten hobbie, an old favorite sport.

Sometimes we must step back, examine our lives and habits, and question our answers. Sit down, close your eyes, and think about the habits you will change. Be ready to make minor and major adjustments. Expect obstacles and breakdowns. But keep going—the reward will be there for you.

Keep in mind that this book is not anybody's final answer. It is work in progress.

As we wrote at the beginning of this book, it is about moderation.

Better keep yourself clean and bright; you are the window through which you must see the world.

—George Bernard Shaw

Bibliography

Alexander CM, et al. NCEP-defined metabolic syndrome, diabetes and prevalence of coronary heart disease among NHANES III participants age 50 years and older. *Diabetes.* (2003). 52:1210-1214.

Boden G, Shulman GI. Free fatty acids in obesity and type 2 diabetes: defining their role in the development of insulin resistance and beta-cell dysfunction. *Eur J Clin Invest.* (2002, Jun). 32 Suppl 3:14-23.

Brand-Miller J, Hayne S, Petocz P, Colagiuri S. Low-glycemic index diets in the management of diabetes, a meta-analysis of randomized controlled trials. *Diabetes Care.* (2003, August). 26(8):2261-2267.

Bray GA, Lovejoy JC, Smith SR, DeLany JP, Lefevre M, Hwang D, Ryan DH, York DA. The influence of different fats and fatty acids on obesity, insulin resistance and inflammation. *J Nutr.* (2002, Sep). 132(9):2488-2491.

Burke JP, Williams K, Narayan KM, Leibson C, Haffner SM, Stern MP. A population perspective on diabetes prevention: whom should we target for preventing weight gain? *Diabetes Care.* (2003, Jul). 26(7):1999-2004.

Despres JP, Lamarche B, Mauriege P, Cantin B, Dagenais GR, Moorjani S, Lupien PJ. Hyperinsulinemia as an independent risk factor for ischemic heart disease. *N Engl J Med.* (1996, Apr 11). 334(15):952-7.

Ferrannini E, Haffner SM, Stern MP, Mitchell BD, Natali A, Hazuda HP, Patterson JK. High blood pressure and insulin resistance: influence of ethnic background. *Eur J Clin Invest.* (1991, Jun). 21(3):280-7.

Ford ES, et al. Prevalence of the metabolic syndrome among US Adults: findings from the third national health and nutrition examination Survey. *JAMA.* (2002). 287:356-359.

Ginsberg HN. Executive summary of the third report of the national cholesterol education program (NCEP) expert panel on detection, evaluation, and treatment of high blood cholesterol in adults (Adult Treatment Panel III). *JAMA.* (2001, May 16). 285(19):2486-97.

Haffner SM. Epidemiology of type 2 diabetes: risk factors. *Diabetes Care.* (1998, Dec). 21 Suppl 3:C3-6.

Haffner SM, Stern MP, Hazuda HP, Mitchell BD, Patterson JK. Cardiovascular risk factors in confirmed prediabetic individuals. Does the clock for coronary heart disease start ticking before the onset of clinical diabetes? *JAMA.* (1990, Jun 6). 263(21): 2893-8.

King H, Aubert RE, Herman WH. Global burden of diabetes, 1995-2025: prevalence, numerical estimates, and projections. *Diabetes Care.* (1998, Sep). 21(9):1414-31.

Knowler WC, Barrett-Connor E, Fowler SE, Hamman RF, Lachin JM, Walker EA, Nathan DM: Diabetes Prevention Program Research Group. Reduction in the incidence of type 2 diabetes with lifestyle intervention or metformin. *N Engl J Med.* (2002, Feb 7). 346(6):393-403.

Lindstrom J, et al. Prevention of diabetes mellitus in subjects with impaired glucose tolerance in the Finnish diabetes prevention study: results from a randomized clinical trial. *J Am Soc Nephrol.* (2003, Jul). 14(7 Suppl 2):S108-13.

Meigs JB. Epidemiology of the insulin resistance syndrome. *Curr Diab Rep.* (2003, Feb). 3(1):73-9.

Moller D. *Insulin Resistance.* (1997). Chichester: John Wiley and Sons Ltd.

Ovalle F, Azziz R. Insulin resistance, polycystic ovary syndrome, and type 2 diabetes mellitus. *Fertil Steril.* (2002, Jun). 77(6):1095-105.

Pi-Sunyer FX. The obesity epidemic: pathophysiology and consequences of obesity. *Obes Res.* (2002, Dec). 10 Suppl 2:97S-104S.

Reaven GM. Banting lecture 1988. Role of insulin resistance in human disease. *Diabetes.* (1988, Dec). 37(12):1595-607.

Reaven G, Segal K, Hauptman J, Boldrin M, Lucas C. Effect of orlistat-assisted weight loss in decreasing coronary heart disease risk in patients with syndrome X. *Am J Cardiol.* (2001, Apr 1). 87(7):827-31.

Reaven GM. Importance of identifying the overweight patient who will benefit the most by losing weight. *Am J Med.* (2002, Dec 30). 113 Suppl 9B:38S-40S.

Sahelian Ray. *Be Happier Starting Now: The Complete Mind-Body Guide to Becoming Your Best* (1995). Longevity Research Center Inc.

Smith SC Jr. Review of recent clinical trials of lipid lowering in coronary artery disease. *Am J Cardiol.* (1997, Oct 30). 80(8B):10H-13H.

Tanasescu M, Hu FB. Alcohol consumption and risk of coronary heart disease among individuals with type 2 diabetes. *Curr Diab Rep.* (2001, Oct). 1(2):187-91.

Index